The Perimenopause & Menopause WORKBOOK

A Comprehensive, Personalized Guide to Hormone Health for Women

KATHRYN R. SIMPSON, MS
DALE E. BREDESEN, MD

New Harbinger Publications, Inc.

Publisher's Note

Care has been taken to confirm the accuracy of the information presented and to describe generally accepted practices. However, the authors, editors, and publisher are not responsible for errors or omissions or for any consequences from application of the information in this book and make no warranty, express or implied, with respect to the contents of the publication.

The authors, editors, and publisher have exerted every effort to ensure that any drug selection and dosage set forth in this text are in accordance with current recommendations and practice at the time of publication. However, in view of ongoing research, changes in government regulations, and the constant flow of information relating to drug therapy and drug reactions, the reader is urged to check the package insert for each drug for any change in indications and dosage and for added warnings and precautions. This is particularly important when the recommended agent is a new or infrequently employed drug.

Some drugs and medical devices presented in this publication may have Food and Drug Administration (FDA) clearance for limited use in restricted research settings. It is the responsibility of the health care provider to ascertain the FDA status of each drug or device planned for use in their clinical practice.

Distributed in Canada by Raincoast Books

New Harbinger Publications, Inc.
5674 Shattuck Avenue
Oakland, CA 94609
www.newharbinger.com

Cover design by Amy Shoup; Text design by Michele Waters-Kermes; Acquired by Melissa Kirk;
Edited by Jasmine Star

Library of Congress Cataloging-in-Publication Data

Simpson, Kathryn R.
The perimenopause & menopause workbook : a comprehensive, personalized guide to hormone health / Kathryn R. Simpson and Dale E. Bredesen.
p. cm.
Includes bibliographical references and index.
ISBN-13: 978-1-57224-477-1
ISBN-10: 1-57224-477-1
1. Perimenopause—Popular works. 2. Menopause—Popular works. 3. Middle-aged women—Health and hygiene—Popular works. I. Bredesen, Dale E. II. Title. III. Title: Perimenopause and menopause workbook.
RG186.S6686 2006
618.1'75—dc22

2006026813

08 07 06

10 9 8 7 6 5 4 3 2 1 First printing

To my father, Albert Roland, whose courage in the face of his own progressive neurological disease inspired me to seek solutions.

—Kathyrn R. Simpson

To Aida, Marion, Diane, and the many like them who have suffered through years with untreated symptoms; and to Tara and Tess, who hopefully never will.

—Dale Bredesen

Contents

	Acknowledgments	vii
	Preface	ix
	A Word of Caution	xii
	Introduction	1
CHAPTER 1	It's Up to You: Managing Your Hormone Health	8
CHAPTER 2	Your Health History: Assessing Your Overall Health and Your Family's Health History	28

CHAPTER 3	What's Going On? Assess Your Hormone Balance	49
CHAPTER 4	Out of Balance: Estrogen and Progesterone Lose Their Balance	69
CHAPTER 5	Out of Control: Thyroid Imbalance	89
CHAPTER 6	Out of Steam: Adrenal Imbalance	112
CHAPTER 7	Out of Hormones: Menopause	137
CHAPTER 8	What's Right for You? Bioidentical Hormone Replacement Therapy	152
	Conclusion	179
APPENDIX A	Symptoms at a Glance	181
APPENDIX B	Blood Levels of Estrogen and Progesterone from Various Products	218
	Resources	221
	Recommended Reading	223
	References	225
	Index	239

Acknowledgments

Thanks!

As are all fun and worthwhile efforts, this book was a collaborative project, and thanks must go to Debbie Merino, Jo Ann Roland, Hiram French, Ann McDonald, Jasmine Star, Madeleine Berenson, Marian Lever, Liz Widdicombe, Melissa Brewster, Linda Powell, Ian Blumenthal, Tory Babcock, Anita Chambers, Ann Blumenthal, Margarita Lupin, Kathryn Imani, Kim Rosenstein, MD, and all the doctors and women who were willing to share information and experiences.

And, as always, thanks to our families, Bob, Tyler, Kyle, and Myles Simpson and Aida, Tara, and Tess Bredesen.

Preface

Almost everything that you do, from thinking to growing to emoting to bearing children, is dramatically affected by hormones. Therefore, knowing your hormones and managing them—their levels, their effects, how to optimize them—and being familiar with the symptoms of hormone imbalance are as important as anything else you do for your health. Proper nutrition and exercise are certainly important, but even the best nutrition and exercise regimen will do little to correct the symptoms of hormone imbalance. If you're tired or depressed, have difficulty shedding pounds, or have irregular menstrual cycles, then you have symptoms suggestive of hormone imbalance.

Over the last few decades, we as a nation have focused on health issues from cholesterol to blood pressure to diet and exercise. And we have reaped the rewards.

As a society, we're living longer, healthier lives and doing more than ever before. We're no longer surprised when we hear of someone in their seventies or eighties completing a triathlon or starting a new company. But hormone health hasn't received the attention given to vitamins, diet, and exercise. This is somewhat surprising, since vitamin deficiencies are relatively uncommon in our society today, whereas hormonal effects are typically much more striking than the effects of vitamin supplements. So, in a sense, hormones are the new vitamins.

However, we don't yet know the optimal doses of either vitamins or hormones. For vitamins, we have an RDA, or a recommended daily requirement, but no guidelines for optimal daily intake. In fact, we don't know how much vitamin C, A, or B_6 is best for us, and the picture emerging for hormones is much the same: We have general guidelines for "normal" levels of each hormone, but as of yet we simply do not know the "perfect" level for each hormone. And to make matters more complicated, this level will probably turn out to be different for each person. What this means in practical terms is that managing your hormones is based on a combination of comparing your levels to the "normal" levels and then carefully monitoring your body's response to therapy. The effects of doing this can be absolutely remarkable on your health, and the number of healthy years in your life. This workbook, easy to read and easy to follow, will help you with every aspect of your hormones, from recognizing the symptoms of hormone imbalance to understanding the function of various hormones to finding the right doctor and getting the right treatment.

I have been fortunate to work with lead author Kathy Simpson, an absolutely remarkable woman. After years as a successful businesswoman, Kathy developed multiple sclerosis (MS). Voracious reading and studying led her to conclude that hormonal imbalances were contributing to her MS. Sure enough, it turned out that she did have such imbalances, and since she has corrected these she has had no further MS attacks nor disease progression—and her symptoms have all resolved. Although it is virtually impossible to prove that correcting her hormonal balance was in fact directly responsible for her marked clinical improvement, recent research supports a connection between hormone balance and MS. Higher estrogen levels (such as those that occur with pregnancy) are associated with a reduction in multiple sclerosis attacks, and this may be mediated by estrogen's effect on the immune system's T-regulatory cells (Polanczyk et al. 2004).

Kathy has now been symptom-free for three years. She is youthful, vivacious, active, and absolutely committed to helping as many people as possible to understand, manage, and optimize their own hormonal health. She and thousands of others are proof that hormones have dramatic effects on energy, weight gain, response to stress, and so many more health parameters. She's "been there and done that"—she has firsthand experience with many of the symptoms described in this workbook—and no medical degree can substitute for personal experience with symptoms. Therefore, her background is perfectly complementary to my own in clinical and research medicine. Together, we have tried to create a book that will be perfect for you, a book that will give you exactly what you need to manage one of the most critical aspects of your health and your life.

So, we invite you to read on. Completing this workbook is easier than navigating the Internet, easier than following an exercise and nutrition regimen, and easier than juggling family and career. You can do this! And, believe us, it *will* be worth it!

—Dale Bredesen, MD

A Word of Caution

Our intent is to share knowledge and information based on our personal experience and available scientific research. The information in this book is not intended to replace the care of a physician or other licensed health care professional, nor is it intended as medical advice. If you have symptoms or suffer from an illness or health condition, you should always consult with a qualified health professional to accurately analyze and diagnose what is going on.

We believe strongly that all women are individual in their physical makeup and situations, and no two women will have the exact same set of health conditions, making it impossible to understand what the correct treatment path will be for any given woman without individualized testing and evaluation under the care of a trained health professional.

It is important to understand that anyone who wishes to embark on any dietary, drug, exercise, or other lifestyle change intended to prevent or treat a specific disease, condition, or symptom should first consult with the appropriate health care professional, and no treatment should be initiated or stopped (particularly any prescription drugs you may be taking) without this medical supervision.

Introduction

At forty-three, after months of struggling with fatigue, bladder problems (five bathroom visits a night was too many), hair loss, irregular menstrual cycles, and numbness in my hands, I finally made an appointment with my doctor to see what was going on. He listened to my list of woes then referred me to four other doctors: a urologist for my bladder problems, a neurologist for my numbness, a dermatologist for my hair loss, and an ob-gyn for the irregular bleeding. As for the fatigue, he told me, "You have three young children, of course you're tired!"

I asked whether it might be perimenopause and whether there were any tests we could do. "Don't be silly," he said. "You're too young for that!" Like most women over forty, I like hearing anyone say I'm too young for anything, but this didn't help me with my physical problems. I was also dismayed by the urologist's advice: "I can't find anything wrong. This just happens to women your age. You're going to have to get used to it." And the neurologist's: "It's carpal tunnel syndrome. You need surgery." And the ob-gyn's: "You're still having your period, so your hormones are fine." By then, I couldn't face one more doctor, so I didn't even bother with the dermatologist. The idea that my only option was to get used to it—in other words, stay within fifty feet of a bathroom, take afternoon naps for the rest of my life, and undergo surgery on my hands—left me feeling completely discouraged.

In the meantime, my symptoms were worsening. Midcycle bleeding became a monthly problem. I had trouble concentrating and remembering even everyday words, my hair started falling out in earnest, and I was exhausted all the time. So, a few months later, I went back to my ob-gyn. This time he did some testing—not for estrogen or progesterone levels but for follicle stimulating hormone (FSH, a hormone that increases when estrogen levels start to decrease). He discovered that my readings were nearing the menopausal range and recommended birth control pills to even out my cycle and regulate the bleeding. I filled the prescription and went home hoping that this would take care of everything. Unfortunately, the medication made me feel worse. After two months I stopped taking it, and I was back to square one.

Over the next two years, I went into a frightening downward spiral. With no clear medical solution, I did the only other thing I could think of: I changed my diet and became a strict vegetarian. I ate mostly pasta and vegetables and did what everyone was doing at the time—cut out meat and fats. I learned the hard way that my reasoning, and diet, were faulty. My cholesterol level dropped to 120 from 200, and I began to feel even worse. (I know now that some hormones are made from cholesterol, so lowering my levels so drastically only aggravated my situation.) The numbness spread to the side of my face, I started to lose vision in my right eye, and all of my other symptoms got worse.

I went back to the neurologist. After a five-minute consultation, he said, "You have multiple sclerosis" and scheduled a spinal tap to confirm the diagnosis. Unfortunately, the spinal tap site "leaked" afterward (not an uncommon occurrence, I later learned), and as my neurologist had left town on an untimely vacation, I had to lie flat and couldn't raise my head over the level of my spine for over a week without crushing pain. This insult to my central nervous system launched a whole new set of symptoms, including almost complete loss of vision, generalized muscle spasms, and widespread numbness. Even more unfortunately, the test was positive for multiple sclerosis (MS).

I came through it, though, more determined than ever to regain control of my body and my health. Having worked as the director of operations for a large biotech firm, and having managed various pharmaceutical research and development projects, I'd seen incredible advancements in science and medicine firsthand. This experience, combined with my determination to get my health back, convinced me that if I took the research into my own hands, I could get to the bottom of what was happening. So I sat down one night, made a list of all the symptoms I was experiencing, and Googled every one. And guess what? They all came back "hormones." Bladder control? Hormones. Fatigue? Hormones. Hair loss? Numbness? Unusual bleeding? Hormones. Fussy? Tired? Impaired vision? Hormones, hormones, hormones!

I spent the next few months learning everything I could about hormones. I read books and spent hours and hours on PubMed—the online research site of the National Institutes of Health. Then I picked up the phone and called Dr. Dale Bredesen, a colleague and friend (and coauthor of this book), who is CEO of the Buck Institute, one of only five nationally recognized centers of excellence in research on aging in the United States. Dale is a leading expert in the field of aging and its associated diseases, so when he didn't think I was crazy, I knew I was on to something. Then I went back to my doctor. This time I was armed with both confidence from my intensive research and the resolve to take responsibility for my own health. I badgered, cajoled, and coaxed him into writing me a prescription for estrogen and progesterone. I felt certain that hormone replacement therapy (HRT) was a potential solution for me. He finally wrote the prescription, and that's when I started to get my life back. The last piece of the puzzle fell into place when I added thyroid and adrenal therapy a couple of years later.

Today as I write this, I'm sitting in my office with a full head of hair and excellent vision in both eyes (I don't even need my reading glasses anymore!). I can go for hours without having to find a bathroom, and I have more than enough energy and enthusiasm to manage my career and my three sons, and to put renewed energy into my marriage—something my husband of thirty years appreciates. I still have some numbness in my right hand, but I feel certain it would have been reversible as well if I had started on the hormones sooner.

You can see why I'm incredibly passionate about hormones. My life and health have been profoundly affected by them, first negatively by multiple deficiencies, and then positively by their replacement. I've spent the last two years working with Dale, researching and organizing the information to write this book. If what I've learned can spare other women unnecessary anxiety, fear, and discomfort, or help them have the confidence and clarity to become experts in their own bodies so they can seek appropriate care and the treatment they need, this will have been a challenge worth enduring.

It may have been difficult for you to pick up this book. Hormone imbalance, perimenopause, menopause—these are names of clubs we don't want to belong to. Acknowledging that this is the stage of life we are in, or soon will be, isn't easy for most of us. Women in their early thirties have trouble believing hormonal change or imbalance is affecting them, but more and more women are experiencing perimenopause at that age. No matter how young or old we are, it seems most of us would rather not think about it. We'd rather stay young, act young, feel young, be young. That's exactly why we've written this book. We believe wholeheartedly that aging doesn't have to mean feeling old, tired, feeble, weak, or sick. We believe that the more we know about ourselves and our bodies, and the more responsibility we take for our health, the greater our chances are of aging with grace, vitality, and joy.

We've chosen to write a workbook because we believe the lists I made when I began researching my symptoms were an important step in organizing and clarifying what was going on with me. When you take a moment to jot down your own personal information in each chapter, you'll be taking that important first step, too.

WHY HORMONE BALANCE MATTERS TO YOU

There isn't a woman among us who doesn't have questions and concerns about how her body is aging and how it's affecting her life. It doesn't matter if you're twenty-five or fifty—hormone imbalance can hit you at any age. All women should be informed about hormone issues and be prepared to understand and manage any slight, or not so slight, hormonal shift.

There are fifty-three million women in this country between the ages of thirty-nine and fifty-three. We're growing faster than any other group, as a percent of overall population. Our health issues differ from the rest of the population. For instance, more and more women are developing cancer, autoimmune diseases, heart disease, Alzheimer's, and depression, as well as experiencing a reduced quality of life. Could these all be hormonally related?

There's no reason to suffer either the symptoms of hormone imbalance or the diseases it can lead to; you can't afford to passively sit by when it comes to your health. For me, the answer to restored health was bioidentical hormones—estrogen, progesterone, thyroid, and cortisol. For you it may be all or none of these, and that's something you can start to figure out by completing the questionnaires and tests outlined in the following pages. It takes some work to get to the bottom of what's going on, but once you do, you'll have a clear picture of any hormone imbalances and deficiencies you may have and how to correct them.

This workbook will guide you through a comprehensive evaluation to help you identify what's happening in your body and what imbalances may be affecting your health and day-to-day well-being. Step-by-step guidelines and questionnaires will help you focus on your health history and your family's health history and symptoms. Hot flashes may be the poster child of menopause, but there are dozens of other symptoms that you might not realize are due to hormonal imbalance and from which you may have suffered unnecessarily. We developed this workbook by integrating an enormous body of peer-reviewed research to address all these symptoms, explain why they're happening to you, and tell you what you can do about them.

Before you can take control and begin making the necessary changes on the path to optimal health and well-being, you need to have an accurate portrait of your hormonal status and health, and this book provides the structure to do just that. The workbook can be used to develop a self-help program and as an aid in working with a health practitioner. It will offer you a clear guide to understanding exactly what bioidentical hormones are and how they work. The distinction between bioidentical hormones, which are identical in every way to the hormones produced in our bodies, and the hormone products that have been widely marketed in the past is extremely important to understand and will be explored in depth.

Some women suffer such serious hormone imbalances that they can't function. The stress they experience and the strain it creates on relationships can cause them to lose friends, jobs, spouses, and even family. Those who say that menopause is a natural process and that all women should go through it naturally (without hormone replacement) ignore the fact that a large percentage of women over the age of fifty in the United States are prescribed pharmaceutical products to cope with their symptoms. Antidepressants or cholesterol-lowering drugs aren't more natural than bioidentical hormones, nor will they usually address the root cause of the problems you may be struggling to cope with.

Your symptoms and well-being are critical elements in this decision process, but there are other, less obvious health indicators that are just as important. You need to have a complete physical: How are your cholesterol levels and blood pressure? Are you insulin resistant? Have you had your bone density measured? Some conditions that can undermine your future health can be prevented, corrected, or reversed by starting hormone therapy early. The bottom line is that the best health choices are made by a woman who thoroughly understands herself and her options. This book is designed to help you achieve that kind of understanding.

HOW TO USE THIS WORKBOOK

This workbook is the product of a long and close collaboration with Dr. Dale Bredesen. We have pooled our experience: Dale's many years of cutting-edge aging research and clinical practice and my personal experience of almost every symptom of hormone imbalance imaginable, along with many years of hormone research and countless hours spent interviewing doctors as well as other women suffering similar symptoms. We've included quite a few case histories to give you an idea of what other women have experienced, and I've also included several pertinent personal stories under the heading "What I Learned" to differentiate them from the stories collected from other women. We hope that this will provide you with a comprehensive and unique perspective on what's happening to your body (or what may start happening in the future). In the interest of simplicity, we've written this book in the first person, but Dale's voice and medical expertise are behind every word.

We believe it's important to have an understanding of the whole picture of hormone imbalance before trying to focus on specific problems, so we recommend that you initially read this book from cover to cover, completing all the questionnaires as you go. Afterward, you can refer back to areas of special interest. We focus on four main areas of potential hormone imbalance: estrogen and progesterone imbalance, thyroid imbalance, adrenal imbalance, and menopause. Some of these issues and imbalances will be new to many of you, and it's difficult to know which you may be suffering from until you've completed the questionnaires and evaluations. You may be surprised by what you find.

After you have completed your initial reading and worked through all of the exercises, you'll be prepared to focus on specific areas of concern that this process has uncovered. Use the table of contents to guide you to the appropriate chapters and the index to help focus your search. If you have unusual symptoms that your doctor isn't familiar with, consult appendix A, Symptoms at a Glance, which is a compendium of most of the hormonal symptoms we've encountered. Don't let it intimidate you. Many of these symptoms are fairly esoteric, and you may have never even heard of them, let alone experienced them. I had many peculiar symptoms (the feeling of bugs crawling on my skin, a symptom referred to as *formication*, to name just one) that none of my doctors had heard of, and which they swore were not hormonally related. Well, they were, and they're all gone now. It's a huge relief to find out that what's been troubling you has a name and a definable cause—and that you're not crazy after all.

You'll need to keep a journal while you're reading this workbook. Consider using a loose-leaf notebook so that you can remove pages to photocopy and share with your doctor. We've provided space to fill in some responses, symptoms, and personal data, but most of the time you'll need a place to write your responses, as well as any additional thoughts or ongoing symptoms as you become aware of them. This is important because it's easy to lose sight of changes that occur over stretches of time—particularly if they're for the better. When you implement diet, lifestyle, and especially hormone therapy changes, you should keep an accurate record of the differences in how you feel. We're certain that once you understand how your hormones work, what can go wrong with them, and how to fix anything that has gone wrong, your diary will be filled with exciting and promising developments.

Here's to your good health!

—Kathy Simpson

CHAPTER 1

It's Up to You: *Managing Your Hormone Health*

Have you ever wondered about the famous glow of a pregnant woman? Is there something beyond the joy of impending motherhood that causes radiant skin, shiny hair, and strong, healthy fingernails? Indeed there is: estrogen and progesterone. A pregnant woman's body is flush with both hormones. But when you're running low on these hormones, you feel the opposite of glowing—tired, dry, irritable, and depressed. Low levels can also cause you to lose interest in sex, even if you're under forty-five or maybe even thirty-five. These symptoms affect your emotional and physical well-being, and they can happen to any of us.

Although it's human nature to ignore things that aren't causing problems, you shouldn't ignore the physical changes that signal hormonal changes going on beneath the surface. If you don't take action until you're plagued by obvious symptoms of hormone imbalance, like hot flashes, you'll have a lot of catching up to do, made all the more difficult if you're hampered by things like brain fog, fatigue, and insomnia. No matter how old you are, understanding your hormones and how they interact with each other is vitally important.

HORMONE BASICS

Hormones work as messengers in your body. These biochemical substances travel through your bloodstream taking messages to all parts of your body, telling your cells what to do, regulating all of your body's functions and keeping everything in constant communication. Hormones are part of the endocrine system, and it's called a system for a very good reason: All of our hormones work together and affect one another, so a dysfunction or imbalance with one often affects many others. In this book, we're mostly concerned with *sex hormones*—those made in the ovaries, such as estrogen, progesterone and testosterone—as well as hormones made in the thyroid and adrenal glands.

Hormones are essential to maintaining your health as you age, and they connect all the parts of your body in ways that would probably surprise you. Has your back or a leg been bothering you? It probably never crossed your mind that this could be triggered by hormones. Most of us would go to an orthopedist and get X-rays or an MRI. We might start physical therapy or even contemplate back surgery. Few of us would consider getting our hormone levels tested. But research has proven that when estrogen, progesterone, and sometimes thyroid hormone levels drop too low, a nerve in the lower back starts to cause pain in the back and often the legs, and exercise or surgery won't help (Kyllonen et al. 1999; Koenig, Gong, and Pelissier 2000).

It's bad enough when we start to see the first physical signs of aging: dry skin, wrinkles, and dull, thinning hair that starts sticking up in odd little peaks and resists styling. But even worse, while we're struggling with these changes, all of a sudden everything and everyone seems to be behaving differently—sometimes almost unreasonably. Or is it us? Guess what? It is us, or rather, it's our hormones. Changing hormone levels can make us emotional wrecks, just like they did when we were teenagers. Do you find yourself muttering, "I'm getting upset over things I would have laughed at last year. I can't even remember the last time I had a good laugh. I hate my husband. I hate sex. What I need is a massage. I want to run away. To Bali. By myself!" But even if we're miserable, we don't want to admit that something is awry with our hormones, the very source of our femininity and fertility. We live in a culture of youth, and it's hard to admit, even to ourselves, that our hormone levels may be changing.

If this is starting to happen to you, you may feel as though there's nowhere to turn. Your doctor says, "It couldn't be your hormones: You're too young, you still have your period, you're just tired, and why wouldn't you be? You work full-time, you have young children, you have teenagers," and so on. Then you get the inevitable prescription to take a vacation, antidepressants, or birth control pills. But these don't seem to help, and you don't know what else to do.

It might help to know that you're not alone. There are about forty million menopausal women in the United States today, with twenty million more baby boomers entering, or already in, perimenopause (U.S. Census Bureau 2005). Unlike previous generations, we have the wonderful opportunity to really understand what's going on with our hormones. The good news is that this doesn't have to be a painful process. You can educate yourself and be prepared for what's to come. You don't have to be taken by surprise. You don't have to be at the mercy of startling symptoms. You don't have to end up feeling bad, or looking bad. You have a choice. By completing this workbook, you're taking the first step in assuming control of your own health and hormones.

FIVE CRITICAL HORMONES

The word "hormone" comes from the Greek word *hormon*, which means "to stir up." Think back to puberty (or just this morning if you're in perimenopause) and you can see where this came from. Understanding various hormones and what they do will put you in a much better position to understand what your symptoms mean and what tests are necessary to identify and correct them. Here's a basic overview of the five most critical hormones that are affected as you age: estrogen, progesterone, thyroid hormones, cortisol, and testosterone (Marieb 2001).

Estrogen

Estrogen is sexy, fertile, strong, happy, and voluptuous (with lots of hair and beautiful skin). The Dolly Parton of hormones, estrogen is known as the "female hormone" because it plays a key role in shaping the female body, particularly the breasts and hips, and preparing it for uniquely female functions, such as pregnancy. In addition, the vagina, uterus, and other female organs depend on the presence of estrogen in the body to mature.

Estrogen (along with progesterone) plays a critical role in your monthly menstrual cycle and prepares your uterus for pregnancy. More than 90 percent of the estrogen in a woman's body is made by the ovaries, with other organs (including the adrenal glands, liver, and kidneys) making the rest. At menopause, the ovaries markedly decrease their estrogen production, but low levels are still produced in these other organs, as well as in fat cells. This is why women who are overweight when going through menopause may have fewer problems with symptoms related to lack of estrogen, such as hot flashes and vaginal dryness. Our bodies make three major types of estrogen: estradiol, estrone, and estriol.

Estradiol is made in the ovaries. This form of estrogen makes you youthful, fertile, agile, and smart. Necessary for almost every function in the body and brain, it triggers growth of neurons and cells and is responsible for all those things you want to keep as you age: good memory and a sharp mind; great sex drive; plenty of energy; a cheerful, calm outlook on life; clear, smooth skin; and ideal weight. When the ovaries shut down at menopause, the only way to get more estradiol beyond the minimal amount made by the adrenals is through hormone replacement (C. J. Gruber et al. 2002). *When I use the word "estrogen" in this book, I'm referring to estradiol unless otherwise noted.*

Estrone takes over after you stop making much estradiol at menopause. It's produced mainly in your fat cells and liver. The more fat you have, the more estrone you make. Unfortunately, estrone blocks estradiol action, so you may start to have symptoms of estrogen deficiency as you gain weight. Estrone doesn't have any of estradiol's antiaging abilities, such as maintaining skin, hair, and bone. It has also been proven to increase your risk of early heart attack, diabetes, and reproductive cancers.

Estriol is produced in high levels only during pregnancy and doesn't play a part in our perimenopausal and menopausal story.

Progesterone

Youthful, cheerful, calming, steady, well-balanced, and fertile, progesterone is the Goldie Hawn of hormones. Formerly thought to be just the pregnancy hormone, it was named for "pro-gestation," but researchers have since found progesterone receptors all over the body, indicating that progesterone has wider functions. (Receptors allow the body to receive and utilize hormones, and once a hormone attaches to its receptor, it causes specific chemical changes in the body.) Areas with progesterone receptors include the reproductive tract, urinary tract, heart, blood vessels, bones, breasts, skin, hair, mucous membranes, pelvic muscles, and brain (Nash, Morrison, and Frankel 2003).

Progesterone is made primarily after ovulation by the empty egg sac after it has released an egg. So when you don't ovulate, you make much less progesterone, throwing off the delicate balance between estrogen and progesterone. An ovulation tester, which can be purchased at any drugstore, should be part of every thirty- and forty-something woman's arsenal. It provides an easy way to keep tabs on whether you're ovulating or not, clueing you in to the first signs of hormonal imbalance.

Thyroid Hormones

Your thyroid is the epicenter of your body, connecting, communicating with, energizing, and regulating everything to keep you in order. Think Oprah Winfrey. Your thyroid gland is a critical component in overall hormone health, just as Oprah is in the communication of women's issues. This gland is responsible for regulating all metabolic functions in the body, which is not just about how we digest food and whether we gain weight. The thyroid controls all energy production and use in the body—every tissue, every cell. If your brain isn't working well, your libido is gone, or your hair is falling out, it could be due to low thyroid function. The list of symptoms of low thyroid function makes a compelling case for its importance: Fatigue, accelerated aging, weight gain, joint and muscle pain, dry skin, constipation, memory loss, brain fog, and hair loss are just a few of these symptoms. And since thyroid function is closely intertwined with other hormones, such as cortisol, estrogen, and progesterone, thyroid dysfunction affects their ability to function, as well.

Cortisol

Cortisol gives you energy, helps you handle stress, and enables you to be quick and active. It's the vibrant, enduring Tina Turner of hormones. Cortisol is produced in the adrenal glands, which become increasingly important as you age. As the ovaries' production of estradiol and progesterone slows, the adrenals become the backup producers for these critical hormones.

Considered a "stress hormone," cortisol is produced when you perceive a threat to your well-being or survival. It's produced by any stressor, from not having enough food to being chased by a lion. When the increase in cortisol levels is of short duration, our memory works better, we have more energy, and we're more motivated—all critical to getting out of the path of that charging lion (or for Tina when she's on stage). Unfortunately, if you're under stress for a long period of time and your cortisol level remains elevated, it becomes toxic, causing depression, memory malfunction, stressed-out behavior, loss of energy, and other negative effects. When your adrenals finally get exhausted by all this frenzied cortisol production, you'll become even more tired, find yourself feeling cold all the time, get allergies you never had before, lose your stamina, have blood sugar regulation problems (resulting in weight gain), and ache all over.

Testosterone

With her beautiful teeth and bones, muscle tone, sex appeal, coordination, drive, and fantastic energy, Madonna is the personification of good testosterone balance for a woman. Testosterone is one of several hormones referred to as *androgens*, or "male hormones," and although we typically think of men when we think of testosterone, it's also an important hormone for women, especially for building muscle mass and bone. Testosterone has also been found to have a significant effect on libido, mood, and energy. There are testosterone receptors in most areas of the body responsible for sexual function, including the nipples, vagina, and clitoris, so it's easy to see why dropping levels can result in decreased libido and sexual function. By age forty, levels of testosterone drop to half of what they were at twenty and continue dropping. Testosterone is made mainly in the ovaries, like estrogen and progesterone, so when our ovaries stop producing hormones at menopause we finally lose much of our supply.

Hormones work together in our bodies like a close-knit team. Everyone's there—Dolly, Goldie, Oprah, Tina, and Madonna. They all have very distinct, important characteristics (sex appeal, balance, health, energy, and ability to handle stress), but the interactions among them are equally as important and one can't function without the others. When all are present in the right proportion, we are our most balanced and healthy selves. Later in this chapter we'll take a look at some common hormone imbalances, but first let's take a look at how women's hormones optimally function during our reproductive years.

THE MENSTRUAL CYCLE

The menstrual cycle is a finely tuned and choreographed process of fertility. The beginning of your cycle, or day one, is when your body sloughs off the uterine lining from the previous cycle and your period begins. The first half of the cycle is the follicular phase; the second half is the luteal phase.

The follicular phase is the time in which the *follicles*, or eggs, ripen for potential fertilization, leading up to ovulation at about day fourteen. Progesterone is very low throughout this time, as is estrogen, until around day five. Then estrogen levels increase dramatically to a crescendo at ovulation, when the egg is released from the ovary for fertilization. During this last week leading up to ovulation, we are happy and mentally alert, our hair shines, our athletic abilities are never better, and our sex drive is at its peak. This makes sense, as these qualities help guarantee the continuation of the species: High estrogen levels ensure that we're at our most responsive at the time of ovulation, when it's easiest to get pregnant, and that we're at our most alluring when we need to attract a partner to accomplish this goal.

The luteal phase is the second half of the cycle and lasts about two weeks. It's named for the *corpus luteum*, the empty egg sac left behind after the egg is released at ovulation, which produces the estrogen and ever-increasing levels of progesterone necessary to ready the uterus to receive the fertilized egg. Progesterone is critical to balance the estrogen produced in the first half of the month, as it stops the cell proliferation caused by estrogen. It also makes some women feel foggy, sluggish, and clumsy. These symptoms are much worse if your estrogen level starts to decline while you're still ovulating, because your estrogen levels should also rise pretty dramatically at this time to balance your escalating levels of progesterone. Assuming you don't become pregnant during the cycle, progesterone peaks around day twenty-one and then starts to decline. This triggers your uterine lining to start shedding a week later, resulting in your period.

The following graph shows the varying blood levels of progesterone and estrogen during a normal menstrual cycle.

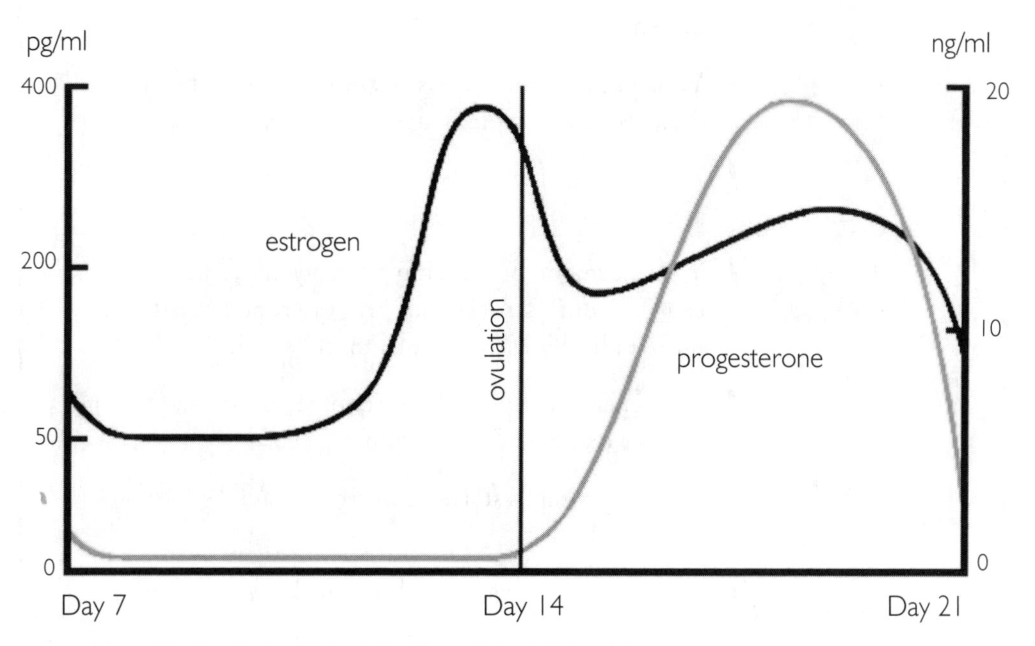

Estrogen and Progesterone Levels in the Menstrual Cycle

Not only do your hormones change cyclically every month with your menstrual cycle until you reach menopause, they also change over the course of your reproductive life. The following table shows some changes you can expect every decade or so.

Hormonal Changes by Decade	
In your twenties	Estrogen production and fertility usually peak at age twenty-seven to twenty-eight and then start to decline slowly.
In your thirties	You no longer ovulate every cycle. When this happens, you don't make progesterone in the second half of the cycle, which estrogen to be overly dominant and un-balanced. Your progesterone levels begin to decrease fairly dramatically at around age thirty-five. Your estrogen level also starts to decrease more rapidly after thirty-five.
In your forties	Your hormone production becomes more imbalanced, causing your estrogen and progesterone levels to vary more radically within your monthly cycle. Your menstrual periods start to get irregular (either shorter or longer in duration). Your egg supply starts to decrease, causing further estrogen loss. You experience cycles with no ovulation more often. Thyroid disorders become much more common.
In your fifties	Your estrogen, progesterone, and testosterone levels are very low and progesterone eventually drops to almost nothing when you reach menopause. Your thyroid function is greatly affected by loss of estrogen and progesterone, as the thyroid glands have ovarian hormone receptors and vice versa. Your menstrual cycle generally stops in your early fifties (fifty-one is the median age), but it can happen much sooner or, for a very few, in the late fifties.

FOUR COMMON HORMONE IMBALANCES

If you're reading this book, you're probably already suffering from symptoms of hormonal imbalance. The following are four of the most common hormone imbalances women experience. In chapters 4 through 7, I'll cover each of these in detail. If your symptoms are interfering with your life, or if the descriptions below sound scary or unpleasant, don't be discouraged; although I once had most of these imbalances, I'm now completely healthy and symptom free at fifty-two.

Out of Balance: Estrogen and Progesterone

As you age, your levels of estrogen and/or progesterone drop, with one often decreasing more rapidly than the other. When this happens, their finely tuned balance can be thrown off and cause unpleasant symptoms and health problems.

Estrogen loss: Some women, particularly those who are slim and small breasted, have biologically lower levels of estrogen. If you're one of these women, when your hormone levels start to fall estrogen often gets too low for your body to function at its best. As a result, you may experience symptoms such as bladder problems, hot flashes, difficulty concentrating, loss of sex drive and function, mood swings, irritability, and conditions such as osteoporosis, as early as your late thirties or early forties. If your progesterone levels remain high during this time, the added imbalance caused by high progesterone in relation to your low estrogen levels may result in additional symptoms, such as depression, drowsiness, and headaches. If this occurs well before the onset of menopause, don't be surprised if your doctor tells you that you're too young for hormones to be the cause of your symptoms. (Of course it sounds great to be thought too young for just about anything, but don't let it deter you from finding out what's really going on.) Doctors rarely diagnose early imbalances correctly, so remember that the only way to detect an imbalance is to measure your estrogen and progesterone levels. If you have any or all of the above symptoms, you may have low estrogen levels and you may want to consider estrogen replacement.

Progesterone loss: For many other women, the slowing of progesterone production, not estrogen, is the first sign of hormonal imbalance. This usually occurs in the mid-to late thirties, when ovulation becomes irregular and fails to produce enough progesterone to effectively balance estrogen levels. If this happens, it's important to detect and resolve it quickly, because excess estrogen in relation to progesterone is associated with many unpleasant and potentially dangerous symptoms: uterine fibroids, insomnia, fibrocystic breasts, anxiety, weight gain, fatigue, excessive bleeding, and even breast cancer. Even though your estrogen level may be "normal," if your progesterone is low, you're in an excess estrogen state. Excess estrogen also suppresses thyroid function (Furlanetto et al. 2001). And without healthy thyroid function, your adrenals (where cortisol is made) can't function properly, so you start to experience symptoms such as weight gain, fatigue, and concentration problems.

Out of Control: Thyroid

Your thyroid gland is in charge of all metabolic activities and controls the functioning of every single cell in your body. This means that if your thyroid malfunctions, *every* cell in your body suffers. Your thyroid makes hormones that increase the amount and activity of mitochondria (those little energy generators in each cell), which convert what you eat into body heat and energy. So when your thyroid isn't functioning well, you may feel cold and tired and gain weight. This is one of the easiest problems to solve. If your thyroid hormone levels are low, thyroid replacement can resolve these symptoms. Unfortunately, thyroid function tests are notoriously inaccurate when it comes to detecting low thyroid, so thyroid malfunction is often overlooked and misdiagnosed. Because of this, you must look carefully at your symptoms and see if a pattern of low thyroid appears. Use this to guide you, and your doctor, to an accurate diagnosis and treatment.

On the other hand, a small percentage of women have overactive thyroids, which causes opposite symptoms, such as hyperactivity and weight loss. This condition, if left untreated, may result in loss of thyroid function, ultimately causing symptoms of low thyroid.

Out of Steam: Adrenals

If your adrenals either overwork or stop functioning well, it's a major problem, as your adrenals are critical to good health. They're responsible for producing several key hormones, including cortisol and adrenaline, which, among other things, control how we manage physical and emotional stress, or the fight-or-flight response.

It doesn't matter whether you're experiencing either good stress, such as excitement, or bad, such as pressure or trauma; in either case your adrenals are mobilized and cortisol production is ramped up. This stress response sends a burst of energy that helps you survive life-threatening situations, which in the past generally involved fighting or fleeing from hostile tribes or carnivorous beasts. But even if the challenge in front of you is less traumatic than a charging lion, your body still goes through the same physiological changes to send immediate energy to your muscles. At the same time, your heart rate, breathing rate, and blood pressure increase to provide more oxygen and nutrients. Other, less critical body functions, like digestion, hormone production, tissue repair, sex drive, and immune function are slowed since they aren't critical to the perceived emergency at hand.

You can see how taxing all this ramping up and mobilizing can be to your body. Think how debilitating this would be if it didn't stop once you'd escaped the charging lion. But this is precisely what happens to you after years of being bathed in cortisol from ongoing stressors, such as a frustrating boss, escalating house payments, and babies (or teenagers) that don't sleep. It makes sense that you'd run out of stored energy and start to feel tired a lot of the time, get sick more often, and even overreact to minor stressors you used to handle easily.

To compound the demands on your adrenals, cortisol not only manages your body's response to emotional and physical stress, it also regulates the effects and interactions of other hormones in your body. If your adrenals are fatigued, they can't effectively do everything they should, so they must prioritize what gets done and what doesn't. Unfortunately, producing and managing hormones takes a backseat to survival.

Rebalancing or rebuilding your adrenals takes a concerted effort. But a quick review of the symptoms caused by adrenal malfunction should convince you it's worth it: extreme fatigue, difficulty exercising, muscle and joint aches, hypoglycemia, alcoholism, anxiety or panic attacks, allergies, asthma, and more frequent or severe infections.

Out of Hormones: Menopause

This final hormonal shift is a big one: At menopause, your ovaries drastically reduce production of estrogen, progesterone, and testosterone. You may be one of the lucky few who makes it through this menopausal transition full of vim and vigor, happy to be free from menstrual cycles and the responsibilities of pregnancy and raising children. But for most of us, it isn't a joyous time. It takes a bit of effort to accomplish the transition smoothly as we shift from production of estrogen and progesterone in our ovaries to the much lower backup supply of hormones produced by our adrenal glands.

Women tend to take physical complaints in stride, buck up, and keep right on going. We put our families first, and ourselves and our health on the back burner. We've also experienced a history of not being taken seriously and being accused of having mysterious emotional complaints. In the past, the medical community lumped these complaints into the "female hysteria" category and offered us medications for anxiety and depression, thinking our symptoms were psychosomatic. In fact, the word "hysteria" literally means "wandering uterus," as the thought was that only women could have such complaints. We know now that what's going on is physical and not psychosomatic, and we see the consequences of hormonal imbalance and deficiency in our friends and family members, manifested in the ever-increasing incidence of conditions that used to occur only in old age: osteoporosis, weight gain, chronic fatigue, and even cancer.

THE IMPORTANCE OF BASELINE TESTING

If some of the imbalances and symptoms described above seem to apply to you, you may be wondering how you can find our what's going on. The very best way is to test your hormone levels. In an ideal world, your estrogen, progesterone, and other hormone levels would have been tested when you were a young woman so that you'd have baseline information on what's normal for your body. You would know what levels your body naturally produces and functions best with. Think about it this way: Unless you know that 98.6°F is a normal temperature, how would you know when you have a fever, or that you need to treat it? It's the same with hormones: You need to establish baseline hormone levels to know how far your imbalance swings above or dips below your norm.

There are no right or wrong levels—your own personal level and balance is what's important. But unless you had your hormones tested before they were seriously out of whack, which is unlikely, you won't know what your body is used to, or at what levels you feel best. We can help our daughters take a different path, but for

Fat Phobia Can Harm Your Health

In the 1980s, the United States was swept with "fat fear." Fat would give you heart disease, high cholesterol, and even cancer. Diet books and the media were full of the theory that the vast majority of the fat on your body came from the fat you ate. This has since been disproved, but it is so deeply ingrained in many of us that we have a hard time using butter or any other fat liberally. (Certainly, if you consume enough fat you can get fat, but this is true of consuming large quantities of almost any food.)

We now know that dietary fats are necessary for many critical functions, including manufacturing hormones. Your ovaries require a certain amount of fat to make estrogen, progesterone, and testosterone. You may be surprised to learn that cholesterol, that much-maligned and feared substance, is what your body uses to make these steroid hormones. If you don't have enough cholesterol, you may find your levels of these key hormones dropping, accompanied by all the symptoms of low hormone levels. This has widespread implications at the cellular level, because hormones are necessary to make new cells and break down old ones. They're also necessary for facilitating your body's assimilation of fat-soluble vitamins. (So if you're taking fat-soluble vitamins, such as A, D, E, and K, you need to take them along with a meal containing some fat so that they'll be absorbed effectively.)

Clearly, fats are a very important ingredient in your diet, but as with everything else in life, it's important that you don't overdo it. Americans currently get 40 to 50 percent of their calories from fat—somewhere in the neighborhood of sixty-nine pounds per year (Putnam 2000). A more balanced and healthy amount would be no more than 30 percent.

most of us, who didn't know to check our levels when we were young, we're in the position of trying to deduce what our levels were. One clue is that most of your hormone status is inherited, the way you inherit nose size and eye color. You're born with a genetically programmed plan to produce high, low, or average levels of estrogen and progesterone. Believe it or not, your body's shape will give you a good idea of what your inherited levels are, and the most important factor offering a visual clue of your estrogen level is the size of your breasts (although breast development can be affected by other factors as well).

WHAT YOU SEE IS WHAT YOU'VE GOT: HORMONES AND YOUR BODY'S SHAPE

A clinical study at a European university was conducted to determine if there was a correlation between breast size and estrogen and progesterone levels. Breast size, along with a waist-to-hip ratio that creates the classic hourglass figure, is one of the primary, biologically programmed measures men use to judge female attractiveness. The study proved that large breasts and a narrow waist are indeed an external sign of fertility, and that women with these physical characteristics do have higher levels of estrogen and progesterone than other women, and thus greater fertility. Lab tests showed that these women had 26 percent higher overall estrogen levels, with 37 percent higher levels at ovulation (Jasienska et al. 2004).

Of course, many of us are more average physically, with bodies that indicate neither obviously high nor obviously low estrogen levels. This indicator that your levels are in the midrange also suggests your potential path through perimenopause and menopause. The good news is that because your levels aren't especially high, you won't have such a large potential drop when your ovaries do stop producing estrogen, so you shouldn't experience dramatic symptoms. Because you have fairly robust levels of estrogen production, you're less likely to run out prematurely and experience significant impact from symptoms of low estrogen, such as vaginal and bladder discomfort.

Effects of Higher Estrogen Levels	Effects of Lower Estrogen Levels
You have significantly larger breasts.	You have smaller breasts.
You're relatively short (high levels of estrogen make bones "close" and stop growing).	You're relatively tall because your bones continued to grow for a longer period of time.
You feel worse when your estrogen level begins to drop with age.	Your estrogen levels drop earlier because you had less estrogen to begin with.
You're more likely to have excess estrogen in relation to progesterone.	You're more likely to have excess progesterone if you continue to ovulate after your estrogen drops.
You feel much better when progesterone is added to balance your higher levels of estrogen.	You feel much better when estrogen is supplemented.
You feel worse if estrogen is added before you complete menopause; even the low amounts of estrogen in birth control pills can cause you to feel worse.	You feel worse if progesterone is added while you're still ovulating.
You're more likely to experience symptoms of excess estrogen, such as sore breasts, heavy periods, excessive bleeding, and development of fibroids.	You're more likely to experience symptoms of low estrogen, such as severe hot flashes, bladder problems, and dryness of the vagina, skin, hair, eyes, and mucous membranes.

EXERCISE: Assessing Your Inherited Estrogen Level

Take a minute to think about your body type and those of your mother, sisters, grandmothers, and aunts. In your journal, list all of your female blood relatives' names, and for each, jot down indicators that might give you a clue as to your inherited estrogen level, such as height, breast size, and response to any hormone-containing therapies (for example, birth control pills or fertility drugs) you or your relatives have taken.

Lori's Story

Lori, fifty-three, is short with large breasts and an hourglass figure, indicating a high genetic level of estrogen. Her mother and sister are also short and buxom. Her mother developed fibroids (growths in the uterus generally caused by too much estrogen relative to progesterone) and experienced very heavy and prolonged bleeding in her late forties, which resulted in a hysterectomy. She was then put on the horse-derived estrogen product Premarin, which she remains on today—twenty years later.

In her midforties, Lori did what most of us do: She gained weight. But she also suffered other hormone imbalance symptoms, including insomnia, mood swings, fatigue, memory problems, anxiety, and depression. Her doctor prescribed antidepressants, which helped a bit with her depression but didn't affect her other symptoms.

Lori realized she wouldn't be able to keep up with her family and job without relief from her symptoms, so she started to read everything she could about women's health and aging. The information she uncovered convinced her that hormones were the root cause of what she was experiencing. She talked with her mother and found that she had many of the same symptoms that had resulted in her mother's hysterectomy: excessive bleeding and pain with her periods, which signaled the possible development of fibroids. After finding a doctor willing to measure all of her hormone levels, Lori discovered that her estrogen measured 300 pg/ml (picograms per milliliter), a higher level than many women have at age twenty. At the same time, her progesterone level was "undetectable."

Her thyroid hormone levels were also very low, suppressed by the high levels of estrogen untempered by adequate progesterone.

Lori's imbalance between estrogen and progesterone was undeniable, and her doctor started her on an over-the-counter progesterone cream. This didn't seem to have any effect at all, so several months later her doctor agreed to start her on prescription-strength progesterone. Many of her symptoms resolved immediately, and after a couple of months she felt her equilibrium return. Under her doctor's supervision, Lori gradually weaned herself off the antidepressants. Her weight also started to drop without any change in her diet, and when she had her thyroid hormone levels measured six months later they were completely normal, showing the dramatic effect that balancing her estrogen had on her thyroid function.

Susan's Story

Susan is skinny, with small breasts. She had two children, her first at thirty-five and the second at thirty-nine. In order to conceive, she had taken the fertility drug Clomid (clomiphene), which works by hyperstimulating the ovaries to produce more egg follicles, thus increasing the odds of conception. But producing more egg follicles means eggs deplete faster. And since estrogen is produced by follicles and maturing eggs, fewer eggs also means less estrogen production.

By her midforties, Susan had problems with incontinence whenever she sneezed or laughed, but it never crossed her mind that hormones might be causing the problem. Then her eyes started getting very dry and her vision worsened noticeably. She noticed an overall feeling of dryness and not just in her skin and hair—even sex was uncomfortable as vaginal dryness started making intercourse difficult. She had no idea what was causing these symptoms, but it wasn't until she started to miss periods that she went to her ob-gyn.

Her doctor measured her estrogen level at only 30 pg/ml—in the menopausal range—and started Susan on bioidentical estrogen and progesterone replacement consisting of oral estrogen and oral progesterone.

The effect was immediate: Dryness was no longer a problem, and her bladder problems resolved within the first month.

Although it's a relatively good indicator, body type alone doesn't tell us everything. And, of course, many of us fall somewhere between the two distinct types exemplified by Lori and Susan. So no matter what your physique, if you'd like to manage perimenopause by maintaining healthy hormonal balance, you've got to look deeper. You need to understand the common imbalances, evaluate your symptoms, and test your hormone levels. And regardless of where you fall on the estrogen and progesterone spectrum, the best strategy for optimizing your health and hormone balance will include a healthy diet and an active lifestyle.

PERIMENOPAUSE

The period of time in which the balance of your hormone levels starts to change is known as *perimenopause*. It may start in your thirties or forties, and it will continue until you reach the final stage, menopause, probably sometime in your fifties. Contrary to popular belief, menopause is not a single event waiting to devastate your life, nor is it the same experience for every woman; it's a highly individualized transition. Perimenopause is a natural phase of life, though sometimes a difficult one. It's when you don't understand what's happening and don't know how to manage it, or even that you *can* manage it, that your health, and even your sanity, can be challenged.

The first order of business in understanding and managing this transition is to complete your health history. Chapter 2 will guide you through developing both a personal and a family health history. Use this as a catalyst to call your mother, sisters, grandmothers, aunts, and, if you're lucky enough to still have them, great-grandmothers. Talk with them about their health and their experiences with hormonal issues and record what you find out. All of this information will help you start to build an accurate and comprehensive picture of your genetic inheritance. It will also tell you what conditions or diseases you need to be on the lookout for and what kind of preventive measures you should take.

Things to Remember

- Physical changes and symptoms that result from shifts in hormone levels and balance may also signal that potentially more serious health conditions are occurring (for example, osteoporosis or heart disease).
- Hormone levels may start to drop fairly drastically in your midthirties.
- Four of the most common hormone imbalances and deficiencies involve hormones produced in your ovaries (estrogen and progesterone), your thyroid gland, and your adrenal glands (cortisol).
- Breast size is a good general indicator of inherited estrogen levels and can be used to anticipate your path through perimenopause. If you have large breasts, it's more likely that you'll experience symptoms and conditions associated with high estrogen and deficient progesterone. If you have small breasts, you're more likely to experience symptoms of low estrogen.

CHAPTER 2

Your Health History: *Assessing Your Overall Health and Your Family's Health History*

Debbie's Story

Debbie started to have minor, irritating health problems in her late thirties. When she was thirty-eight, the first health concern that triggered a doctor's visit was increasing patches of raised, scaly, reddish skin. Her skin had gotten drier and drier over the last several years, but this was something new. She went to a dermatologist, who said the condition looked like psoriasis and gave her a topical ointment. She faithfully applied the ointment, but it seemed to have no effect and the patches continued to itch. The next symptom Debbie noticed was seasonal allergies: In the spring the trees in her backyard had her sneezing and blowing her nose, and then she noticed that if she didn't wash her hands after petting her cat, her eyes would swell up and water if she touched her face. She became sensitive to smells and chemicals that never used to bother her.

In her early forties, Debbie was told at a routine physical that her cholesterol levels indicated an increased risk of heart disease. Her overall level was 189, but her "bad" cholesterol (LDL) was very elevated at 150, and her "good" cholesterol (HDL) was too low at 39. Her levels of triglycerides (fat in the blood), at 152, were also high, increasing her risk of developing heart disease. Her doctor told her that with this cholesterol profile, she needed to seriously try to lose the thirty extra pounds she had slowly gained in the last few years.

Debbie left her doctor's appointment determined to get her weight under control and lower her cholesterol levels. Unfortunately, it wasn't easy. She went on a low-carbohydrate, high-protein diet and lost seven pounds in the first two weeks. But when she went off this severely restricted diet all the weight came back, and she seemed to be getting even thicker through the middle.

At forty-nine, she began to suspect that her current, worsening health issues were the cumulative effect of ten years of not fixing the underlying problems. This spurred her to try a new approach. She went to a wellness clinic, where the first course of business was completing a health history questionnaire and undergoing a thorough physical exam. The health history indicated to her doctor that hormones were most likely at the root of her varied and continued health problems, so he ordered lab tests including levels of estrogen, progesterone, thyroid hormones, and cortisol. The results indicated that she had a serious thyroid deficiency, complicated by adrenal deficiency. All her symptoms, starting with psoriasis (Leslie and Levell 2004), allergies, and chemical sensitivities and ending with weight gain and increased risk of heart disease, were indicative of low thyroid and adrenal function.

Debbie started on prescription thyroid hormones combined with low-dose cortisol therapy to rebuild her adrenals and felt much better almost immediately. Her psoriasis also started to respond quickly and within several months had completely disappeared.

GETTING TO THE BOTTOM OF YOUR HEALTH PROBLEMS

As you can see from Debbie's story, sometimes the seemingly minor exercise of filling out a health history can be the key to discovering the cause of confounding and long-term health problems. So as you work through the checklists below, think about every issue in each category carefully. Don't brush off any symptoms you've experienced as "not that bad" or "not worth mentioning." It's an unfortunate fact that women tend to neglect their own health and try to ignore any symptoms or discomfort they're having as long as they can. But compiling your health history gives you a chance to get a reading on how your body is functioning, what is causing you concern, and what in your history may be the catalyst for these symptoms. Record as much detail as you can about each health issue. This will be a vital tool when working with your doctor to get to the bottom of the symptoms you're experiencing.

Take your completed health history with you when you meet with your doctor. It's impossible to collect your thoughts while you're filling out forms in the waiting room. You can't possibly remember all the important details while desperately trying to complete the questionnaire so as not to lose your place in the queue, let alone think through if there might have been a hormonal catalyst for any of the conditions you do remember to write down, or some other connection that might be the key to a long-standing health problem. We all know how frustrating it is to wait and wait for a scheduled appointment only to remember while driving home a critical piece of information that we forgot to tell the doctor.

Don't be embarrassed to bring in all the information needed to fill your doctor in on every detail of your history. Doctors are only as good as the information you give them and most appreciate all the help you can provide. If you find a doctor who's reluctant to listen or is uninterested in your information, it would probably be best to look for a doctor who will enter eagerly into this process with you.

EXERCISE: Health History Checklist

Read through the symptoms in the following list and check any that apply to you, whether now or in the past. Use the checklist to trigger memories of other health conditions and events; for instance, if you check "excessive menstrual bleeding," you may then remember that after this started you had to have an endometrial biopsy.

CARDIOVASCULAR/HEART

- ☐ Ankle swelling
- ☐ Blood clots
- ☐ Chest pain or pressure
- ☐ Heart disease
- ☐ Heart murmur
- ☐ High blood pressure
- ☐ High LDL cholesterol
- ☐ High triglycerides
- ☐ Irregular heartbeat
- ☑ Light-headed spells
- ☐ Mitral valve prolapse
- ☐ Phlebitis
- ☐ Valvular disease

EYE, EAR, NOSE, AND THROAT

- ☐ Allergies
- ☐ Blurry vision
- ☐ Cataracts
- ☐ Change in vision
- ☐ Dry mouth
- ☐ Feeling of fullness in neck
- ☐ Frequent sinus infections
- ☐ Glaucoma
- ☐ Hay fever
- ☐ Hearing difficulties
- ☐ Hoarseness
- ☐ Ringing in the ears or tinnitus
- ☐ Runny nose or congestion
- ☐ Swollen lymph glands

GASTROINTESTINAL

- [x] Abdominal distention
- [ ] Abdominal pain or cramping
- [ ] Blood in stool
- [ ] Bowel incontinence
- [ ] Change in bowel habits or stool
- [ ] Colitis
- [x] Constipation
- [ ] Crohn's disease
- [ ] Diarrhea
- [x] Excessive gas or bloating
- [ ] Heartburn
- [x] Hemorrhoids
- [ ] Hepatitis
- [ ] Irritable bowel syndrome
- [ ] Jaundice
- [ ] Nausea
- [ ] Rectal bleeding
- [ ] Ulcers
- [ ] Vomiting

GENITAL & URINARY

- [ ] Abortion
- [ ] Blood in urine
- [ ] Burning on urination
- [ ] Cervical dysplasia
- [ ] Excessive menstrual bleeding
- [ ] Fibroids
- [ ] Frequent bladder infections
- [ ] Frequent urination
- [x] Infertility
- [ ] Irregular periods
- [ ] Kidney stones
- [x] Low sex drive
- [ ] Menstrual problems
- [ ] Miscarriages
- [ ] Painful periods
- [ ] Pregnancies
- [ ] Sexually transmitted disease
- [ ] Urinary hesitancy
- [ ] Urinary incontinence
- [ ] Urinary urgency
- [ ] Uterus or fallopian tube infection
- [ ] Vaginal infections
- [ ] Venereal disease

MENTAL HEALTH

- [x] Anxiety
- [x] Depression
- [x] Difficulty concentrating
- [ ] Emotional problems
- [ ] Feeling of hopelessness
- [ ] Guilty feelings
- [ ] Hallucinations
- [ ] Hearing voices
- [ ] Insomnia
- [ ] Loss of interest in activities you used to enjoy
- [x] Loss of sexual desire
- [ ] Nervousness
- [ ] Obsessive-compulsive disorder
- [ ] Panic attacks
- [ ] Paranoia
- [ ] Severe stress
- [x] Social withdrawal
- [ ] Tension
- [ ] Thoughts of suicide

MUSCULOSKELETAL

- [x] Arthritis
- [ ] Back pain all the time
- [ ] Back pain only at night
- [ ] Gout
- [x] Joint pain or stiffness
- [ ] Leg pain
- [ ] Muscle weakness

NEUROLOGICAL

- [ ] Difficulty swallowing
- [ ] Dizziness
- [ ] Fainting
- [x] Headaches
- [ ] Loss of sensation
- [x] Memory loss
- [ ] Numbness
- [ ] Paralysis
- [ ] Seizures
- [ ] Stroke
- [ ] Tingling
- [ ] Tremor

RESPIRATORY/LUNG

- [ ] Asthma
- [x] Chronic or prolonged cough
- [ ] Coughing blood
- [ ] Emphysema
- [ ] Shortness of breath
- [ ] Snoring
- [ ] Wheezing

SKIN

- [ ] Acne
- [ ] Alopecia
- [ ] Boils
- [x] Dry skin
- [x] Eczema
- [ ] Lesions
- [ ] Nail changes
- [ ] New moles
- [ ] Psoriasis
- [ ] Rashes
- [ ] Rosacea
- [x] Sensitive to sun
- [ ] Warts

OTHER

- [ ] Change in appetite
- [ ] Change in sleep patterns
- [x] Easy bruising or bleeding
- [ ] Excessive fatigue
- [ ] Excessive hair growth
- [ ] Fever
- [x] Hair loss
- [ ] Intolerance to heat or cold
- [x] Night sweats
- [ ] Radiation treatment
- [ ] Shakiness
- [ ] Sweating
- [ ] Unexplained weight gain
- [ ] Unexplained weight loss
- [ ] Other: ______________________
- [ ] Other: ______________________

SPECIFIC CONDITIONS

- ☐ Addison's disease
- ☐ Alcoholism
- ☐ Anemia
- ☐ Anorexia
- ☐ Bulimia
- ☐ Cancer, breast
- ☐ Cancer, colon
- ☐ Cancer, prostate
- ☐ Cancer, other
- ☐ Carpal tunnel syndrome
- ☐ Celiac disease
- ☐ Chronic fatigue syndrome
- ☐ Cirrhosis
- ☐ Diabetes type 1
- ☐ Diabetes type 2
- ☐ Fibromyalgia
- ☐ Graves' disease
- ☐ Hashimoto's thyroiditis
- ☐ Heart attack
- ☐ Hepatitis
- ☐ Jaundice
- ☐ Lupus
- ☐ Melanoma
- ☐ Ménière's disease
- ☐ Multiple sclerosis
- ☐ Myasthenia gravis
- ☐ Osteoporosis
- ☑ Raynaud's phenomenon
- ☐ Restless leg syndrome
- ☐ Rheumatic fever
- ☐ Rheumatoid arthritis
- ☐ Sarcoidosis
- ☐ Scleroderma
- ☐ Sjögren's syndrome
- ☐ Stroke
- ☐ Thyroid problems
- ☐ Tuberculosis
- ☐ Vitiligo

EXERCISE: Summarizing Your Personal Health History

Of course, there are many aspects to your health situation beyond the symptoms and conditions listed above. This exercise will help you develop a complete summary of your health history and current situation. Take your time with this exercise and complete it as thoroughly as possible, thinking back as far as you can for anything that might have been a catalyst for a particular condition. To help you get started, I've provided a couple of examples for each section. Transcribe the suggested headings into your journal, where you'll have more room to fill in the full details. It may take a while to work through all of the sections of this exercise, and reliving health problems can be draining. Don't feel you need to complete your entire health history in one sitting. Take breaks as you need to; it's fine if you take several days to complete this important task.

DETAILS ON ITEMS IN THE HEALTH HISTORY CHECKLIST

Write down any of the conditions or symptoms that you checked above and list as much detail as you can about your experience: How old were you when it occurred? How long did it last? What treatment did you undergo or what drugs did you take? Was it associated with a disease or with some other event (an accident or surgery, for example)? Think about whether there might have been a hormonal catalyst: For example, did the disease or condition start right after a hysterectomy or a pregnancy, or when you started on birth control pills?

Condition	**Age It Occurred and Duration**	**Treatments**	**Comments**
Depression	*38. It improved after 2 years.*	*Paxil—for 2 years*	*The depression started just after the birth of my second child.*
Insomnia	*38. I still have trouble sleeping.*	*Ambien—still taking*	*This also started right after my son's birth.*

ILLNESSES

In regard to specific illnesses, such as severe colds, flu, sore throats, pneumonia, bronchitis, sinusitis, or mono, note the average number of times you've experienced each per year. Try to recall back as far as you can and add any detail you can remember, including any unusual symptoms. Also note if the number and severity of colds you get has changed for the better or worse and see if you can tie this to any major health event, such as an hysterectomy, menopause, or the development of polycystic ovary syndrome.

Illness	Occurrences per Year	Comments
Sinus infections	*At least one per year since my midforties*	*These days I get a sinus infection whenever I get a cold, and it usually lasts at least a week. The problem's gotten much worse since my midforties, when I started having hormone problems, like hot flashes and sleeplessness.*
Pneumonia	*2005*	*I got a bad cold and sinus infection, but since I was busy at work and couldn't rest, it went into pneumonia.*

INJURIES AND ACCIDENTS

Document all major injuries and accidents you've experienced, or any other conditions causing chronic pain, such as lower back strain. Carefully consider any sports or auto accidents that could have affected your neck; whiplash and physical trauma to the thyroid, located in the front of the neck, can be a catalyst for later thyroid problems. Consider whether your pain or other symptoms due to accidents or injuries has increased at any point you can correlate with hormonal events. Try to recall whether you had any change in your health after this incident and whether you noticed additional symptoms or were diagnosed with any disease or conditions.

Injury or Accident	Date	Resulting Conditions
Serious whiplash from a car accident	*2001*	*I started getting tired a lot, have gained a significant amount of weight, and have more trouble sleeping. These problems have been getting worse in the last year since I went through menopause.*
Back injury from falling off my horse	*1995*	*I have back pain from time to time when I strain my back. It got much worse and more frequent after I started perimenopause.*

SURGERIES

List all the surgeries you've ever had, including dental surgery. Include as much detail as possible about the reason for the surgery. Also include the date of the surgery, its outcome, and any subsequent treatment or medication you had to take due to the surgery. Document whether you were given any anesthesia, whether it was local or general, and if you had any adverse reaction to it. Note any symptoms or changes you observed after the surgery, even if you're not sure they were related to the surgery.

Type of Surgery	Date	Comments
Laparoscopy	*2001*	*For infertility. The doctor was looking for endometriosis but found nothing. No problem with the general anesthetic. Started on fertility drugs (Clomid) and got pregnant.*
Sinus surgery	*1990*	*I had surgery because of recurrent sinus infections. They got better for a couple of years afterward, but now I get one per year again and have to take antibiotics to get rid of them.*

MENSTRUAL HISTORY

Levels of both estrogen and progesterone fluctuate widely during the approximately twenty-eight-day menstrual cycle, as shown in the graph "Estrogen and Progesterone Levels in the Menstrual Cycle" in chapter 1. Every woman has her own unique levels and patterns of fluctuation. Try to remember what your menstrual cycle has been like for the last ten years: Have you always felt better after your period ends, until you ovulate (days five through fourteen)? This is when estrogen production is highest and when you may feel your best. If you're not feeling at your best during this part of your cycle, it may signal low estrogen levels and a need for supplementation, or high levels that need to be balanced with progesterone.

Do you feel better or worse in the two weeks after ovulation (day fourteen) and before your period starts? If you feel worse, this can signal that you didn't ovulate and have too much estrogen relative to progesterone. Do you feel worse right before and during your period? This is the low point of monthly estrogen production. If you have an estrogen deficiency, you'll generally feel worse during this part of the cycle. Many women with otherwise sufficient levels naturally have a low point at this time, which can cause symptoms. Are your cycles of normal length and flow, or are they irregular?

Document everything you can remember, especially any significant changes that have occurred in the last five to ten years. Try to document how you feel or what symptoms you experience during each phase of your cycle: Days one through four are menstruation; days five through fourteen are preovulation; and days fifteen through twenty-eight are postovulation. Consider and list symptoms such as these: heavy flow or clotting, depression or mood swings, sore breasts, food cravings, and the like. (For a more extensive list of symptoms you may be experiencing, review the statements in the Hormone Symptom Evaluation in chapter 3.) Since changes in your menstrual cycle can be very revealing of your hormone status, take as much space as you need to record your symptoms and any other comments or thoughts you have, especially anything you'd like to share with your doctor.

Day of Cycle	Symptoms
1-4	*I get headaches almost every month during my period.* *I get very irritable and tired.*
5-14	*I usually feel best at this time.*
15-28	*My breasts are sore.* *I retain water and get bloated and uncomfortable.*

PREGNANCIES

During pregnancy, the body produces extremely high levels of both estrogen and progesterone. This is one of the reasons women are said to have a special glow and beautiful skin when they're pregnant. Write down everything you can recall about any pregnancies, abortions, or miscarriages. Include any episodes of postpartum depression, which indicates hormonal imbalance (particularly low thyroid function).

Pregnancy Date	Outcome	Related Physical and Emotional Experiences
2002	*Miscarriage*	*It was very traumatic, and my hormones went crazy for months afterward. I was very emotional and tired, my hair fell out, and I had insomnia.*
2004	*Had my son*	*No problems.*

For those of you who have had children or full-term pregnancies, try to remember how you felt in the different trimesters. Did you feel best in the first, second, or third trimester? Did you feel better while you were pregnant than before? This could be an indication that you were chronically low in estrogen and the higher levels you experienced during pregnancy made you feel better. Did you feel worse? This would indicate the opposite—that your body has little tolerance for excess estrogen.

Trimester	Symptoms and Experiences
First	*Felt horrible; I was sick the whole time.*
Second	*Felt great; I had lots of energy and slept well. Felt the best in this trimester.*
Third	*Felt good but tired, and I had a hard time sleeping.*

Have you had infertility problems? If so, document in your journal any fertility treatments you've tried (including drugs) and their outcomes.

DENTAL PROBLEMS OR PROCEDURES

Dental problems have a huge effect on overall health. Please note all dental procedures and conditions you've had, including root canals, gum disease, silver fillings, implants, any bone loss documented by your dentist, receding gums, heightened sensitivity of gums or teeth, and so on. Include the date of any procedures or at least the year. Try to recall if you had any other health issues at these times.

Dental Procedure	Date	Coinciding Health Issues
Root canal	*2001*	*It got infected and I had to have it redone after a year. I was very tired and had foggy thinking a lot more during this time. I've felt much better since it was redone.*

SUBSTANCE USE

The use of alcohol and recreational drugs has a profound impact on overall hormonal health. Alcohol depletes B vitamins, which are necessary for memory function; lowers estrogen levels at earlier ages, bringing on menopause prematurely; increases PMS severity; causes greater brain damage in women than men; has been implicated in greater incidence of miscarriages, stillbirths, premature births, and birth defects; causes more anovulatory (eggless) menstrual cycles, causing infertility and hormone imbalance; and causes menstrual cycle irregularities resulting in variable cycle length and heavier and more painful blood flow. There is also a well-established correlation between alcohol consumption and breast cancer (Boffetta et al. 2006).

Adrenal function can be both a cause and an effect of alcoholism; in other words, adrenal fatigue can cause you to crave alcohol, and overuse of alcohol can cause adrenal fatigue. List all potentially harmful substances you've used (including excessive alcohol consumption or any recreational drugs, like cocaine). Give as much detail as possible on your level and frequency of use.

Substance	Year	Amount Used (times per week and amount)
Wine	*1990-present*	*I usually drink about 3 glasses of wine per night, and sometimes more on weekends.*
Marijuana	*1980-1985*	*I smoked marijuana while I was in college, usually about 4 times per week.*

PRESCRIPTION OR OVER-THE-COUNTER MEDICINE AND SUPPLEMENTS

List all medications or supplements you currently use on a daily or regular basis, including even substances such as aspirin or ibuprofen and vitamins and minerals. Document how much you take, or your dosage for prescription medication, how long you've taken it, and any side effects you may have had. Also consider whether any other symptoms or conditions may have started around the same time you began taking a particular drug or supplement.

Medication	Dose	How Long	Reason for Taking and Side Effects
Armour Thyroid	*60 mg*	*4 years*	*Low thyroid test results*
Ibuprofen	*2 per day every couple of days*	*3 to 4 years*	*Chronic back pain*
Glucosamine	*1,500 mg*	*2 years*	*Joint pain*

After you've completed the sections above, turn to a fresh page in your journal and take some time to summarize all of this information. Review everything you've learned while working with this chapter and note anything that might be important to your doctor. For instance, you may have had many dental procedures such as crowns and fillings, but the root canal you had in 2002 coincided with the beginning of your chronic fatigue. Once you've finished your summary, take a break and reward yourself for taking the time to do this critical work. As soon as you feel refreshed, you can tackle the final task in this important process: compiling your family health history.

COMPILING YOUR FAMILY MEDICAL HISTORY

Compiling your personal health history has probably given you a much clearer picture of your overall health and the types of health problems you've experienced in the past. Perhaps it's allowed you to begin to glimpse some possible connections between your hormonal health and seemingly unrelated symptoms and illnesses. Reflecting on your own health history and symptoms is important, but learning about your family's health history may turn out to be just as critical, especially since it can alert you to be on the lookout for health issues that haven't been a problem for you in the past.

Beth's Story

Beth is short with large breasts, indicating a high genetic level of estrogen. Her two aunts are also short and buxom, and both were diagnosed with breast cancer in their late fifties. Both had mastectomies (no chemotherapy) and are doing well today at ninety-one and ninety-three-years old. They have virtually no grey hair, no decrease in cognitive abilities, and very few of the aches and pains and diseases associated with aging. Their profile is one of very high estrogen.

Beth had significant signs of hormone imbalance starting in her late forties. She was a classic example of high estrogen not properly balanced by progesterone, with symptoms such as fibrocystic breast disease and excessive menstrual bleeding. By the time her doctor figured out what was going on by measuring her estrogen and progesterone levels, she had a serious imbalance that could have led to the same outcome her aunts experienced—breast cancer. Fortunately, her doctor detected the imbalance when she was forty-eight and started her on progesterone supplementation to balance her estrogen.

If you have a first-degree relative (your sister or mother) who had breast cancer before age fifty, your risk for breast cancer is approximately doubled (Colditz, Rosner, and Speizer 1996). Women with breast cancer have a 20 to 30 percent greater chance of having at least one relative with the disease. Sometimes the risk link isn't a defective gene but something more basic, such as familial high levels of estrogen, which, if coupled with inadequate progesterone production, exposes you to more estrogen than is healthy and can cause increased risk of breast cancer (Cowan et al. 1981).

You can see why learning about your family's medical history is so critically important. If Beth had known that unbalanced high estrogen could cause breast cancer and had put this together with her aunts' body type and history of breast cancer, she would have been on the lookout for this imbalance in herself and could have taken the necessary steps to minimize her risk even sooner.

We should all learn about our family medical history and understand the medical legacy we share with siblings, parents, grandparents, and even great-grandparents —as far back as possible. Take time to talk with all of your living relatives, especially the women—your mother, grandmothers, aunts, and sisters. Not only will this give you clues about your own health, the information you compile will be a valuable health legacy for your children, allowing them to understand and be on the alert for any familial health risks you identify.

Though it may be a delicate issue, it's especially important that you ask your female relatives what sort of experience they had during perimenopause and menopause. Though no two women have the same experience, knowing what they experienced will give you an idea of what you might anticipate for yourself. If any of them have had a rough time with hormonal imbalance, knowing this will help you be on the lookout for similar symptoms or conditions. Perhaps you can address these situations sooner and avoid some of the negative outcomes they may have experienced. Sadly, you may find that many of your older female relatives didn't experience perimenopause or menopause "naturally"; it may be that some or all of them had hysterectomies. If this is the case, it's important for you to understand why a hysterectomy was thought to be necessary. Although hysterectomies are still all too common, thankfully we're entering an era where women have many more alternatives for addressing hormonal health and imbalance.

Along with your personal health history, you should bring your completed family history with you when you meet with your doctor to evaluate your hormone health. Most doctors' health history paperwork doesn't include this level of detail, but every single item in the extensive list below has hormonal implications and should be discussed in light of any health issues or symptoms you have had or are currently experiencing. They are of particular interest in assessing hormone health, and some of them may shed light on your risk factors associated with potential hormone replacement therapy (HRT). It may take some time for you to contact all your family members to get all of the information you need for your family history. If you'd like to spread the task out, or if you're experiencing troublesome symptoms that you'd like to understand quickly, you can continue reading and working through the next few chapters as you compile your family health history.

What I Learned

I found out well into my hormone research that all my female relatives on my mother's side had low thyroid function. I hadn't thought to ask, and my mother hadn't thought to mention this fact. We never imagined it could be related to MS, but I've subsequently found that extensive research shows thyroid function is vital to nerve health (which you'll read about in chapter 5). When I came across this research, I got my thyroid hormone levels tested. Mysteriously, they were all normal, because I had a condition called *central hypothyroidism,* which doesn't show up on routine thyroid tests. However, because of my family history and the nature of my symptoms (many of them indicative of low thyroid), I convinced my doctor to give me a prescription for a trial course of thyroid hormones. When I started on thyroid replacement, I got dramatically better and the last of my symptoms of MS disappeared. This family history should have been the first thing I did!

EXERCISE: Family Medical History

For each condition listed below, place a letter identifying any family member who has had the condition or disease (in the past or currently) in the space (M = mother, F = father, B = brother, S = sister, GF = grandfather, GM = grandmother, A = aunt, U = uncle). After you complete the checklist, you can supply further details in your journal.

_________Abnormal Pap smear

_________Adrenal disorder

_________Alcoholism

_________Allergies

_________Alzheimer's

_________Anemia

_________Ankle swelling

_________Anxiety

_________Arthritis

_________Asthma

_________Attention-deficit disorder

_________Autoimmune disease

_________Back pain

_________Bipolar disorder

_________Bladder problems

_________Blood clots

_________Blood disorders

_________Cancer

_________Carpal tunnel syndrome

_________Chemical dependency

_________Chest problems

_________Chronic fatigue

_________Cluster headaches or migraines

_________Colonic polyps

_________Constipation or diarrhea (chronic)

_________Dementia

_________Depression

_________Diabetes

_________Difficulty concentrating

_________Difficulty swallowing

_________Dilation and curettage (D&C)

_________Easy bleeding or bruising

_________Eating disorder

_________Elevated cholesterol or triglycerides

_________Endocrine problems

_________Epilepsy or seizures

_________Eye and vision problems

_________Fibrocystic breasts

_________Fibroids

_________Fibromyalgia

_________Gallbladder disease

_________Hearing problems

_________Heart attack

_________Heart conditions

_________Heart disease

_________Heartburn or reflux

_________Hemorrhoids

_________High blood pressure

_________High LDL or low HDL cholesterol

_________History of radiation or chemotherapy

_________Hypoglycemia

_________Hysterectomy

_________Incontinence (bowel or bladder)

_________Inflammatory bowel disease

_________Insomnia

_________Jaundice

_________Joint pain or stiffness

_________Kidney problems

_________Leg pain

_________Liver disorders

_________Memory loss

_________Menopause (difficult)

_________Menstrual cycle disorders

_________Mental illness

_________Mononucleosis

_________Neurodegenerative disease

_________Neurological disorders

_________Osteoporosis

_________Panic attacks

_________Pelvic inflammatory disease

_________Pneumonia

_________Polycystic ovary syndrome (PCOS)

_________Recurrent infections

_________Respiratory disorders

_________Restless legs syndrome

_________Schizophrenia

_________Sensitivity to sunlight

_________Severe hair loss

_________Shortness of breath (chronic)

_________Sinus problems

_________Skin problems

_________Stomach or gastrointestinal disorders

_________Stroke

_________Thyroid disorder

_________Tobacco smoker

_________Tremor

_________Tuberculosis

_________Ulcers

_________Unexplained weight loss

_________Vertigo, dizziness, or light-headed spells

_________Vocal problems

_________Weight gain or obesity

In your journal, write the name of each relative noted in the list above, then give clarifying details about their medical conditions. For example, if the person had cancer, indicate what type of cancer, the severity, and the outcome. For any of the more generic items in the list (bladder problems, menstrual cycle disorders, and so on), indicate the exact nature of the problem (for example, recurrent bladder infections or irregular menstrual periods). In the case of your female relatives, note if the conditions were pre- or postmenopausal.

When you've finished compiling your family medical history information, consider what risk factors you may have inherited (for breast cancer or diabetes, for example), then list these in your journal.

WHAT DO I DO WITH ALL THIS INFORMATION NOW?

Your personal and family medical history is the most valuable tool a doctor has for accurately diagnosing and treating your hormone conditions and deficiencies. For instance, one hormone imbalance can masquerade as another. If all your doctor knows is that you're experiencing severe fatigue, you may be treated for low thyroid when adrenal depletion is actually the root cause of your problem. In this example, if your doctor knows that you developed insulin resistance, diabetes, or high blood pressure in the past, indicating a prolonged period of excessive cortisol production, it may put your current chronic fatigue in another light. Your doctor may surmise that your adrenals have finally become exhausted.

Since you probably haven't gone to the same doctor your entire life, the only person who has all the necessary historical information is you. Take the information you've compiled in this chapter with you when you go to the doctor, along with your completed Hormone Symptom Evaluation (which you'll work on in the next chapter). Most doctors will schedule at least an hour for a first appointment. Use this time to go over every bit of information you've compiled. Be completely open and frank with your doctor, who will be grateful for the thought and effort you've put into it. Doctors so often have to try to piece together what's going on with incomplete or even inaccurate data. You might even consider sending your summary page, as well as your family history and the Hormone Symptom Evaluation, to your doctor prior to your appointment. This will give you a chance to gauge your doctor's willingness to involve you in your own health care.

Things to Remember

- Don't ignore any unusual or abnormal symptoms or changes in your health. Even fairly minor symptoms can be indicative of hormonal changes or the onset of other health problems.
- Your doctor is only as good as the information you provide. Compile a thorough health history and share this information with your doctor.
- Family health history is important too, giving you clues as to health issues to be on the lookout for in the future.

CHAPTER 3

What's Going On?
Assess Your Hormone Balance

Linda's Story

At forty-six, Linda is feeling better than she has in ten years. She got her teaching degree when she was twenty-two and shortly after started a teaching job and married Bill, who was a sales rep at a large corporation. When they were in their twenties, they were busy and struggling financially. So although they wanted children, they decided to put it off. When Linda turned thirty they realized it was time to start a family, but after almost a year of trying with no success, Linda realized she might need help and went to see her doctor. The battery of tests she and Bill went through came back normal, and they were told to just relax and keep trying. After another six months, both of them started to get anxious. Linda went back to her doctor, and this time he started her on a fertility drug. After another year of trying and a few more visits, Linda's doctor suggested in vitro fertilization. As she was almost thirty-four, she and Bill decided it made sense, and three in-vitro procedures later Linda was finally pregnant.

She delivered a healthy daughter, and three years later she conceived a son, at thirty-nine, with no problem. After her son was born, however, her health began to change. She wasn't able to lose all the weight she had gained. She was exhausted during the day, yet couldn't get back to sleep at night after nursing the baby. Her weight continued to creep up no matter what she did. By the time she was forty-two, she was 35 pounds over her normal weight of 120. Plus, her fatigue was getting worse, and it was getting harder and harder to cope with two young children and a full-time job.

Then she started having more disturbing physical problems, starting with difficult periods. Her bleeding became so heavy that she was constantly afraid she would bleed through her clothes, and her periods were often accompanied by intolerable migraine headaches. Then, one month Linda just didn't stop bleeding. Her doctor did an ultrasound and found several fibroids, benign growths in her uterus, which were causing the bleeding and pain. He said they had to come out immediately. Without really thinking about anything other than stopping the bleeding, Linda agreed to a hysterectomy. It went well, but recuperation took a lot longer than she expected. In the month after her surgery, she started losing a lot of hair, her skin seemed to dry up overnight, and she had her first hot flash. She went back to her doctor, who insisted her symptoms couldn't be a result of the hysterectomy as he'd left her ovaries in. He said they should still be producing plenty of estrogen.

Linda's next two years were miserable. She experienced memory problems and profound depression. She approached her doctor, who prescribed antidepressants. These helped with her sadness and mental confusion, but her other symptoms were getting worse. She often woke up at night covered with sweat; she'd throw off the covers and then be freezing five minutes later. And she was so tense and cranky with her husband that he asked her, half jokingly, if she wanted him to find his own apartment. When she realized how close she was to saying yes, she started asking her friends for help and advice.

Linda was surprised at the input she got once she opened up about her problems. Many of her friends had been through similar experiences, and several were now on various hormone therapies. One friend highly recommended her doctor, so Linda made an appointment with her. The new doctor immediately recognized that Linda's symptoms were hormonal and tested her estrogen, progesterone, follicle stimulating hormone (FSH), and thyroid hormone levels. The tests showed her FSH and estrogen levels to be in the postmenopausal range, her thyroid hormone levels to be low, and her progesterone to be extremely low.

It was a relief to finally get to the bottom of why she had been feeling so bad for years. The doctor explained that her symptoms were caused by a combination of low thyroid and low estrogen and recommended that she start on thyroid medication. The doctor also said that Linda had most likely had a thyroid deficiency for a long time, as it's a common cause of infertility as well as some of the other symptoms she had, such as fatigue, dry skin, and hair loss.

Her doctor also told her that a hysterectomy can interfere with blood flow to the ovaries, compromising estrogen production. She prescribed a bioidentical estrogen patch to use all month long, along with progesterone to take on days fourteen through twenty-eight of her cycle, explaining to Linda that she felt somewhat differently than many other doctors about progesterone use. She said that most doctors wouldn't prescribe progesterone for patients who'd had a hysterectomy and no longer had a uterus, but her belief was that all women who take estrogen should balance it with progesterone, just as our bodies naturally do the last two weeks of every menstrual cycle.

She also explained that the symptoms that Linda had experienced in the years leading up to the hysterectomy—including fibroids, excessive bleeding, depression, and mood swings—were caused when she stopped ovulating regularly and her progesterone levels dropped, leaving her with too much unbalanced estrogen. Linda felt better during her first month on the estrogen and progesterone therapy (combined with thyroid) and her symptoms disappeared—no more hot flashes and she felt happier than she had in years.

HOW HORMONE IMBALANCE BEGINS

Unlike Linda, some women sail through shifting hormone levels and perimenopause easily, experiencing few symptoms of hormone imbalance until a year or two before menopause. Unfortunately, most of us experience quite a few symptoms if we don't educate ourselves and manage this process. Since many symptoms can be related to several different hormonal imbalances, it's important to check levels of most of the major hormones affected as we age: estrogen, progesterone, cortisol, testosterone, and thyroid (these tests are explained in detail in chapters 4 through 6). One of the keys to how severe our symptoms get is how greatly our hormone levels fluctuate. Rapid and drastic fluctuations cause much more discomfort than gradually decreasing hormone levels that remain in the same ratio to one another. Managing hormonal swings early on by measuring and balancing your hormone levels is crucial to a healthy, *even pleasant*, hormonal transition. Even if you're one of the lucky few and have only mild symptoms, you should still get your hormone levels tested as soon as possible so that when your levels do start to change, you'll have an established baseline to compare them to.

Early Signs of Imbalance May Be Subtle

One reason the early phase of hormone imbalance can be so confusing is that many of us don't realize we've stopped ovulating regularly. This causes estrogen to be continually unchallenged by progesterone long before we stop having our periods. Because we still have enough estrogen left to create a period, we don't realize that we've stopped ovulating, so our hormones can start going haywire without us knowing it. Most women don't think hormonal imbalance could be causing their health problems until they have obvious symptoms, like excessive bleeding or hot flashes. If you're still having a fairly regular menstrual cycle, it's unlikely that your doctor will test for these imbalances. Your doctor is likely to assume that if you're still having your period, your hormones are fine and thus probably won't feel the need to test your progesterone and estrogen levels. Instead of letting this defeat or

Premenstrual Syndrome (PMS)

Almost one-third of all women experience some level of PMS, which differs from other hormone imbalances in that it isn't diagnosed so much by your specific symptoms, but more by the time when your symptoms appear and disappear. PMS usually occurs in the two weeks before your period and generally stops when bleeding begins. It often begins at perimenopause (sometime after your midthirties) and gets increasingly severe as you age. The most common symptoms are breast lumps and tenderness, headaches, cramps and pain, fatigue, bloating, fluid retention, weight gain, irritability, forgetfulness, insomnia, anger, depression, and mood swings.

There are two schools of thought about what causes PMS. One subset of doctors believes that PMS is caused by estrogen deficiency and may be exacerbated by progesterone, which is produced in high levels at this time of the cycle (Hassan, Ismail, and O'Brien 2004). Typically, this group prescribes birth control pills or estrogen to resolve PMS symptoms. Another subset believes that PMS is caused by progesterone deficiency and adds progesterone during the last two weeks of the menstrual cycle to balance estrogen and thyroid hormones. The truth is that either may be right; it depends on each woman's unique physiology and deficiencies. The adrenals also play a part in PMS, as they're the backup source for estrogen and progesterone production when the ovaries start to sputter. So if the adrenals are already taxed at this time, they may not produce sufficient levels of estrogen and progesterone. Thyroid abnormalities have also been proven to cause PMS symptoms (P. J. Schmidt et al. 1993; Girdler, Pedersen, and Light 1995), with pituitary hormones, endorphins, and other neurotransmitters sometimes also complicit.

depress you, take this opportunity to educate your doctor. If your doctor doesn't seem open or interested, don't feel frustrated or get too demoralized to continue, just start calling your friends to see if any of them can refer you to a doctor who's open to this path.

Don't let these estrogen and progesterone imbalances go undetected over a long period of time, as they can lead to compromised thyroid or adrenal function or even more serious conditions, such as osteoporosis, cancer, or, as in my case, neurodegenerative disease. The good news is that even if you've taken a wrong turn, you can start monitoring and balancing all your hormone levels—estrogen, progesterone, thyroid, and adrenals—at any point along the way.

Food Cravings

Food cravings are a good example of a subtle symptom of hormonal imbalance. Though you may attribute cravings to lack of willpower, many perimenopausal women suffer from food cravings, which are often due to physiological, not psychological, factors. When progesterone levels aren't sufficient to balance estrogen, your body attempts to fix the situation by producing more progesterone. One of the things it requires to manufacture progesterone is magnesium. Since chocolate is very high in magnesium, chocolate cravings can be your body's attempt to get this mineral. However, chocolate is also high in theobromine, a substance that artificially and dangerously overstimulates your adrenals. If your adrenals aren't functioning optimally, the body craves this boost, but repeated stimulation by theobromine can cause adrenal fatigue, and this can lead to hypoglycemia, or low blood sugar. As a result, you'll probably crave simple sugars and carbohydrates, which can raise your blood sugar levels temporarily and help you feel better for a short time. Unfortunately, it also sets off a chain reaction wherein high blood sugar triggers the release of insulin, resulting in your blood sugar level crashing again. Then you crave more sugar and carbohydrates to bring it back up again.

When levels of aldosterone, another adrenal hormone, are also low, the body loses sodium in the urine in exchange for potassium. This is why you have low sodium and crave salt when your adrenals are depleted. Low levels of thyroid hormones can also be a factor in food cravings (and as you may recall, excessive estrogen in relation to progesterone is a common cause of inadequate thyroid function in perimenopausal and menopausal women). Impaired thyroid function decreases the body's ability to use fats, proteins, and carbohydrates. When the body doesn't get what it needs, it responds with increased appetite and food cravings.

TAKE YOUR SYMPTOMS SERIOUSLY

Like Linda, whose story you read at the beginning of this chapter, many women experience multiple symptoms of hormonal imbalance, even if they misunderstand what's happening and assume the symptoms stem from some other cause. When you're busy with daily life, it's easy to attribute symptoms to something else. You say, "I'm just tired because I've been working too many hours, the house is impossible to stay on top of, the kids' activities are insane, I'm not sleeping well . . ." It's what most women do. You tell yourself, "I'm in my forties (or even thirties), I'm bound to have aches and pains, gain weight, feel weak, start to lose my hair and sex drive, and not be able to sleep well." Then you look for individual solutions for each problem: If you're stiff and achy—pain relievers; if you are depressed—antidepressants; if you gain weight—weight-loss drugs. This is counterproductive. You need to find the root cause of your problems, which will allow you to resolve them.

EXERCISE: Hormone Symptom Evaluation

Filling out the following questionnaire is one of the most important things you can do to bring back or maintain good health. Some of the questions may sound odd or even funny, but they will reveal important signs and symptoms of hormonal imbalances. Your responses will give you and your doctor a full picture of your current, and potential, hormone status. Some of these symptoms may sound like conditions or diseases in their own right. While that may be the case, a more holistic (and effective) way of looking at health seeks the underlying cause for disease. If a hormone imbalance is the ultimate cause of your symptoms, it's unlikely that you'll get any relief until this root cause has been addressed.

The four parts of this questionnaire cover the four most common hormone imbalances. Don't be concerned if the same statement appears in two different sections, as the statement may apply to more than one hormonal imbalance. Read the statements, decide on the level of severity or frequency of each sign or symptom, and circle the number that most accurately reflects how that statement applies to you:

0 = None or never

1 = Mild or occasionally

2 = Moderate or often

3 = Severe or always

At the bottom of each page, total up the points circled and write the page total. Carry these totals forward to the end of each section, and then to the corresponding four sections in "Interpreting Your Results" at the end of the questionnaire. If you have symptoms not covered in this questionnaire, jot them down in your journal and bring them to the attention of your doctor.

Section 1

If you're no longer having a menstrual cycle, skip section 1.

The length of my menstrual cycle has become shorter and my periods are heavier, with a lot of clotting.	0 1 2 3
My breasts get very tender and sore.	0 1 2 3
Sex just doesn't interest me anymore. I do have sex, but it's not satisfying.	0 1 2 3
I have hot flashes.	0 1 2 3
All my clothes feel tighter and my stomach seems larger than it used to, but I haven't gained weight anywhere else.	0 1 2 3
I get very irritable and moody.	0 1 2 3
I'm almost always tired no matter how much sleep or rest I get.	0 1 2 3
My thoughts are getting a little strange. I can't believe what crosses my mind.	0 1 2 3
I'm often anxious or agitated.	0 1 2 3
I get a lot of headaches.	0 1 2 3
I'm getting a lot of yeast infections.	0 1 2 3
I'm gaining weight and nothing I do, diet or exercise, seems to stop it.	0 1 2 3

Page total: ________

My hands and feet feel swollen, and my rings and shoes are tight.	0	1	2	3
I crave certain foods, especially sweets and simple carbohydrates (like white bread).	0	1	2	3
For the first time in my life, I have high blood pressure.	0	1	2	3
I have brain fog.	0	1	2	3
Simple things have become confusing and even overwhelming for me.	0	1	2	3
My PMS symptoms are getting worse.	0	1	2	3
I have a hard time concentrating a lot of the time.	0	1	2	3
I have elevated cholesterol.	0	1	2	3
My back and/or leg aches; I feel a constant pain down my leg.	0	1	2	3
I'm having a hard time getting pregnant.	0	1	2	3
I get heartburn a lot, and sometimes I have pain in my abdomen, my right collarbone, or my back.	0	1	2	3
My ovaries ache.	0	1	2	3
My hands and feet get tingling pins-and-needles feelings.	0	1	2	3
I've started to get acne.	0	1	2	3
I have flaky, red patches on my face.	0	1	2	3
I sometimes feel like I have bugs crawling on my skin.	0	1	2	3
I have weird food cravings, similar to when I was pregnant, but now they're for things like ice, chalk, or starch.	0	1	2	3

Page total: ________

I look much, much older than my age.	0 1 2 3
I have osteoporosis or osteopenia.	0 1 2 3
I've had an abnormal Pap test or have been diagnosed with cervical dysplasia.	0 1 2 3
I wake up often at night and don't feel like I get any deep, truly restful sleep.	0 1 2 3
I've been feeling very sad or depressed, and I don't enjoy the things I used to.	0 1 2 3
I'm getting much more hairy.	0 1 2 3
I seem to get sick a lot and have a hard time bouncing back.	0 1 2 3
I have pain during sexual intercourse and sometimes have vaginal itching and discomfort.	0 1 2 3
I feel light-headed and dizzy, almost like I might faint.	0 1 2 3

Section 1 page total: ________

Total number of points for section 1: ________

Section 2

I've been diagnosed with fibromyalgia.	0 1 2 3
I've been diagnosed with carpal tunnel syndrome.	0 1 2 3
I have ringing or buzzing sounds in my ears.	0 1 2 3
I have chronic constipation.	0 1 2 3
I've been losing a lot of hair. I'm worried I might end up bald.	0 1 2 3

Section 2 page total: ________

The outsides of my eyebrows (toward my temples) are getting much thinner. 0 1 2 3

My fingernails have gotten much softer and thinner. They crack and break much more easily. 0 1 2 3

I have ripples or ridges on my fingernails. 0 1 2 3

I have a lot of aches and pains. I have pains in my joints, hands, and/or feet. 0 1 2 3

I have restless legs at night. 0 1 2 3

I have heart palpitations and skipped heartbeats. It sometimes feels as though I'm having a heart attack or panic attack. 0 1 2 3

I'm gaining weight and nothing I do seems to stop it. 0 1 2 3

I get anxious and agitated. 0 1 2 3

I can't concentrate. 0 1 2 3

Simple things have become confusing and even overwhelming for me. 0 1 2 3

My back and/or legs ache. 0 1 2 3

I'm having a hard time getting pregnant. 0 1 2 3

My hands and feet get tingling pins-and-needles feelings. 0 1 2 3

I feel like I'm going crazy sometimes. 0 1 2 3

I look much older than my age. 0 1 2 3

I've had an abnormal Pap test or have been diagnosed with cervical dysplasia. 0 1 2 3

Page total: 12

I have insomnia.	0 1 2 3
My skin has an overall puffy or "quilted" look; even my back looks puffy. It's not fat but almost like I have a layer of fluid under my skin.	0 1 2 3
My hands and feet are always cold.	0 1 2 3
I'm extremely bothered by heat and/or cold.	0 1 2 3
I seem to have almost no body hair anymore.	0 1 2 3
I have hemorrhoids.	0 1 2 3
I have a chronically low basal body temperature. (See chapter 5 for details on monitoring your basal body temperature for hypothyroidism.)	0 1 2 3
I bruise easily.	0 1 2 3
I get urinary tract infections.	0 1 2 3
I have a weak, soft pulse.	0 1 2 3
I have pain and swelling around my liver.	0 1 2 3
My neck is thickening in the front and I have a lump under my Adam's apple.	0 1 2 3
My face and eyelids are puffy.	0 1 2 3
I have incredibly dry skin, especially on my feet.	0 1 2 3
My vision has become variable. Sometimes one or both eyes have blurry vision and then it gets better.	0 1 2 3
Sometimes I can't hear well out of one or both ears, but after hours, or days, it goes away.	0 1 2 3

Page total: 13

My skin and the whites of my eyes are yellowish and pale.	0	1	2	3
I'm often breathless. It's hard to catch my breath even when I'm not exerting myself.	0	1	2	3
My voice sometimes gets hoarse for no reason.	0	1	2	3
Sex doesn't interest me anymore.	0	1	2	3
I've lost a considerable amount of weight without cutting back on what I eat.	0	1	2	3
I've developed eczema or psoriasis.	0	1	2	3
I've noticed my eyes appear to be swelling or protruding more.	0	1	2	3
The skin on my upper arms and the front of my thighs appears to be getting thicker when I pinch it between my thumb and forefinger.	0	1	2	3

Section 2 page total: ______

Total number of points for section 2: ______

Section 3

I'm not interested in sex.	0	1	2	3
I have symptoms of low thyroid. I tried thyroid hormone supplementation and felt better for a little while, and then I felt worse.	0	1	2	3
I have dark rings under my eyes.	0	1	2	3
I've recently developed asthma.	0	1	2	3
I get cold sweats.	0	1	2	3
I have bowel problems.	0	1	2	3

Section 3 page total: ______

Statement				
I crave sweets.	0	1	2	3
I can't seem to stop drinking alcohol.	0	1	2	3
Sometimes I feel like I'm going to faint.	0	1	2	3
I feel like I'm shaking or shivering inside.	0	1	2	3
I'm irritable and moody.	0	1	2	3
I often have a hard time concentrating.	0	1	2	3
I've become forgetful.	0	1	2	3
Simple things have become confusing and even overwhelming for me.	0	1	2	3
I've started to get many more allergy symptoms.	0	1	2	3
I have a hard time getting going in the morning.	0	1	2	3
I crave salty food.	0	1	2	3
I have environmental sensitivities. Scents like perfume, chemicals, or air pollution bother me.	0	1	2	3
I have respiratory or sinus infections that sometimes last for several weeks.	0	1	2	3
I've experienced chronic stress, or a very significant stressful event, and have felt shaken and not myself ever since.	0	1	2	3
I drive myself constantly and feel like I can never catch up. I feel like I have virtually no time for relaxation and rest.	0	1	2	3
When I introduce people, I panic and forget their names.	0	1	2	3
I seem to get sick a lot and have a hard time bouncing back.	0	1	2	3

Page total: ______

I feel best after dinner.	0	1	2	3
I can't handle stress.	0	1	2	3
I have to drink coffee or other caffeinated beverages to keep going.	0	1	2	3
I often feel guilty or blame others.	0	1	2	3
I often feel tired or depressed, but after eating ice cream or candy I feel much better and happy for a short time.	0	1	2	3
I have abdominal pain or gas.	0	1	2	3
I avoid social engagements.	0	1	2	3
Light bothers my eyes much more than it used to, and I'm uncomfortable when I don't wear sunglasses.	0	1	2	3
I have nightmares.	0	1	2	3
I've noticed that different parts of my body have turned strange colors and/or the creases of my joints appear darker.	0	1	2	3
I can't take a deep breath.	0	1	2	3
When I go to get something, I forget what I went for.	0	1	2	3
When I press on the area of my back at the bottom of the rib cage near my spine, it hurts.	0	1	2	3
I'm gaining weight around my middle section out of proportion to the rest of my body.	0	1	2	3
I'm tired a lot of the time. I crave sweets, white flour products, and chocolate.	0	1	2	3
I have difficulty keeping a job. I get irritated with people I work with.	0	1	2	3

Page total: 16

I'm especially sensitive to color, sound, and odor.	0 1 2 3
When I get up quickly from a reclining position, I get dizzy. Sometimes I black out or everything becomes dim.	0 1 2 3
I get angry easily, which may result in my yelling. It takes a long time to recover.	0 1 2 3

Section 3 page total: 3

Total number of points for section 3: 44

Section 4

When I sneeze or laugh, I leak urine. I'm sometimes uncomfortable from vaginal itching and pain, or I seem to be getting frequent bladder infections.	0 1 2 3
Sex doesn't interest me anymore, and I often find it painful.	0 1 2 3
I have hot flashes.	0 1 2 3
I'm irritable and moody most of the time.	0 1 2 3
I'm often anxious or agitated.	0 1 2 3
I get headaches often.	0 1 2 3
I'm gaining weight.	0 1 2 3
I crave sweets, white flour products, and chocolate.	0 1 2 3
For the first time in my life, I have high blood pressure.	0 1 2 3
I can't concentrate and my memory isn't good.	0 1 2 3
Simple things have become confusing and even overwhelming for me.	0 1 2 3

Section 4 page total: 9

For the first time in my life, I have elevated cholesterol.	0	1	2	3
I feel isolated and don't want to talk to people, or do any of the things I used to.	0	1	2	3
I look much older than my age.	0	1	2	3
I have osteoporosis or osteopenia.	0	1	2	3
I wake up often at night and don't feel like I get any deep, truly restful sleep.	0	1	2	3
I'm told I'm snoring loudly, and I never used to snore before.	0	1	2	3
I've been feeling very sad or depressed, almost miserable, for no real reason.	0	1	2	3
I have dry eyes and have to blink all the time.	0	1	2	3
I have pain during intercourse and sometimes have vaginal itching and discomfort.	0	1	2	3
I've noticed that my gums bleed when I brush my teeth, or my dentist has told me I have larger "pockets" in my gums.	0	1	2	3
My teeth sometimes ache, but when I have X-rays or a dental exam there's nothing wrong.	0	1	2	3
I feel light-headed and dizzy, almost like I might faint.	0	1	2	3
I have a very weak voice. It's getting harder for me to speak up and my voice tires easily.	0	1	2	3
My back and/or legs ache.	0	1	2	3

Section 4 page total: 19

Total number of points for section 4: 28

19
9
8

Don't forget to use your journal to record any other symptoms you're experiencing that don't appear in the sections above. Record any health problems or anomalies you've noticed, even if you're not sure they're hormonally related.

INTERPRETING YOUR RESULTS

Estrogen and Progesterone Imbalance Total number of points for section 1: NA

If your total score is between 10 and 20, you may be in the early stages of perimenopause and should get your levels of estrogen, progesterone, and FSH measured as a baseline. You should also get baseline testing for thyroid and adrenal function.

If your total is between 21 and 50, you have a more significant imbalance between your estrogen and progesterone levels. You should consider purchasing an ovulation tester to determine if you're still ovulating. Also, get your levels of estrogen, progesterone, FSH, thyroid hormones, and cortisol tested.

If your score is over 50, you have significant imbalances and symptoms. You also may have started to develop more serious conditions, like osteoporosis. Have your levels of estrogen, progesterone, FSH, thyroid hormones, and cortisol tested as soon as possible. You also should consider having a thorough physical and a DEXA bone scan for osteoporosis. See chapter 8 for a discussion of treatment options for this hormone imbalance.

Thyroid Imbalance Total number of points for section 2: 39

If your total points are between 15 and 25, you're beginning to show signs of thyroid dysfunction. It's possible you are either hyper- or hypothyroid. Have your thyroid hormone levels tested, along with your estrogen, progesterone, FSH, and cortisol levels.

If your score is over 25, you're most likely experiencing significant thyroid function imbalance (and/or adrenal imbalance as well). Have a complete physical, including a thyroid exam with lab tests. Also have your levels of cortisol, estrogen, progesterone, and FSH tested. See chapter 5 for a discussion of treatment options for thyroid dysfunction.

Adrenal Imbalance Total number of points for section 3: 44

If your total points are between 15 and 25, you may have some level of adrenal dysfunction and should consider a complete adrenal evaluation and cortisol level testing. As thyroid is often involved in adrenal dysfunction, also have a complete thyroid evaluation, including testing of your thyroid hormone levels. Also test FSH, estrogen, and progesterone to get baseline levels.

If your score is between 26 and 40, you're most likely suffering from a significant level of adrenal exhaustion, which is most likely starting to affect the function of other hormones as well. Have all the tests recommended in the previous paragraph done.

If you scored over 40 points, your adrenal dysfunction is potentially severe. Test cortisol levels (as well as all other hormones). See chapter 6 for a discussion of treatment options for adrenal dysfunction.

Menopause Total number of points for section 4: 28

If your total points are over 20, your ovarian production of estrogen and progesterone has most likely diminished significantly. Have your levels of these hormones tested, as well as FSH, thyroid hormones, and cortisol. If you have symptoms that significantly affect your quality of life, hormone replacement options should be discussed with your doctor. See chapter 8 for a discussion of HRT treatment options.

USING WHAT YOU'VE LEARNED

Now that you've completed the Hormone Symptom Evaluation, you should have a much better idea of your hormone status and any imbalances that may be affecting you. If your responses indicate any hormonal imbalances you weren't aware of, schedule an appointment with your doctor as soon as possible so that you can have your levels tested and start working on solutions. The next four chapters will discuss the four main imbalances in detail. Though you'll want to work through all four chapters eventually, if you're having particularly troublesome symptoms of a specific imbalance, you might want to turn to that chapter first.

Things to Remember

- Irregular ovulation is often the first hormonal imbalance you experience. Since there are no obvious signs when you don't ovulate, this can occur for a long period of time and create problems associated with excess estrogen, such as fibroids, without you knowing it.
- Test levels of estrogen, progesterone, FSH, thyroid, and cortisol to see if you have any imbalances, or to help establish your baseline levels.
- Take your symptoms seriously. They'll help you understand what sorts of hormone imbalances you may be suffering from, and then you can work to resolve them.

CHAPTER 4

Out of Balance: *Estrogen and Progesterone Lose Their Balance*

Nancy's Story

At thirty-eight, Nancy was diagnosed with early menopause based on one test result showing elevated follicle stimulating hormone (FSH, the hormone that stimulates ovulation). Nancy didn't have her estrogen or progesterone levels tested. She'd had one son at thirty-five but shelved plans to have a second child after this diagnosis, which was very disappointing as she and her husband had hoped for more children.

In measuring her hormone levels several years later, it turned out that she hadn't been in menopause at all, she'd simply had a cycle without ovulation, which temporarily raised her FSH level. (It's common for the FSH level to rise when your body tries unsuccessfully to ovulate and then return to normal when you ovulate again. For this reason, FSH isn't very reliable for diagnosing hormone imbalances.)

If Nancy's doctor had measured her estrogen and progesterone levels, he could have detected the deficient progesterone that caused her FSH level to spike in that month. If she had supplemented progesterone in the last two weeks of the cycle, Nancy's progesterone levels could have been normalized, restoring her natural rhythm, and her symptoms would have vanished. This misdiagnosis had a profound effect on Nancy, preventing her from having the second child that she and her husband wanted.

THE BALANCING ACT

As you can see from Nancy's story, even minor or sporadic fluctuations in levels of estrogen and progesterone have profound effects on your essential biological functions. Progesterone receptors are found throughout your body in most of the same areas as estrogen receptors (C. J. Gruber et al. 2002), confirming the close, reciprocal relationship between the two. Common sense tells us that the presence of these receptors indicates that both estrogen and progesterone are needed for all these areas to function properly. Progesterone also functions as a precursor, or building block, to many other hormones, including estrogen, cortisol, and testosterone. Together, estrogen and progesterone help to promote and maintain overall hormonal balance.

When your hormone levels start to change, it's important to take action right away because the balance between estrogen and progesterone is critical to maintaining your youthfulness, health, and well-being. Estrogen and progesterone work together in perfect synergy; estrogen tells our cells to grow, grow, grow during the first part of the menstrual cycle, allowing for continual replenishment of old cells with new, and then progesterone steps in to redirect them to develop and die, stopping cell growth. However, for some women progesterone disappears while estrogen is still in a growth mode. When this happens, the resulting excess estrogen causes problems—from relatively minor symptoms such as brain fog, irritability, and lumpy, sore breasts to serious health threats, such as fibroids and endometrial, uterine, and breast cancer (Ansquer et al. 2005).

When the delicate balance of estrogen and progesterone is upset, you start to notice confusing symptoms, such as changing periods, insomnia, weight gain, memory difficulties, and depression. The unfortunate reality is that imbalances between estrogen and progesterone are very common. In your thirties, before you're even aware of such a thing as hormone imbalance, your progesterone levels begin to drop. At the same time, your estrogen levels may start to decline and become erratic. As your body valiantly tries to stimulate ovulation, you alternate between low and high estrogen levels (Prior 2005). This seesaw effect causes problems that are compounded when ovulation sometimes doesn't occur and progesterone isn't produced.

Since estrogen is critical to your feeling of well-being, you might think that the more you produce, the better you'll feel, but actually the opposite is true. In reality, drastic swings in estrogen levels make you feel worse, and they also disrupt progesterone production. It's the *balance* between estrogen and progesterone that's the key to feeling good during this hormone transition. If your estrogen levels decrease gradually and maintain the same ratio to progesterone, you'll have a much easier time and fewer symptoms. When the shift is way out of balance, it generally causes unpleasant symptoms, like irregular menstrual cycles and excessive bleeding.

You're encouraged by your doctor to monitor your cholesterol levels regularly, but I believe it's equally important to measure and monitor estrogen and progesterone levels, since these hormones are just as critical to your health and well-being. All women go through a period of time when these two key hormones fluctuate. With simple blood tests (listed in the "Testing Options" section below) and an ovulation tester, you can measure and balance your hormone levels to prevent unnecessary symptoms. That's right, you can use a simple, inexpensive ovulation test right at home. You don't have to go to a doctor to find out if you're ovulating every month. You can detect anovulatory cycles when they happen and balance your estrogen by supplementing progesterone during those months. By taking charge, you can manage the process instead of letting the process manage you.

Estrogen Levels Drop

You're born with your entire life supply of eggs, which produce most of your estrogen and progesterone. Each time you ovulate, your supply shrinks. You started out life with about half a million eggs, but by your mid- to late thirties you have only five thousand to ten thousand left. Because of this steep decline in remaining eggs, estrogen and progesterone levels start to decrease noticeably in most women at about age thirty-five. This decline continues for the next fifteen years, and by the age of fifty, when many of us have reached menopause, estrogen levels have dropped between 40 and 80 percent (Eskin and Dumas 1995). In thinner women, levels usually drop even lower. As you saw in the graph in chapter 1, most women have average estrogen levels of around 50 to 100 pg/ml in the first two weeks of their cycle, peaking at 300 to 500 pg/ml at ovulation, then dropping to 200 to 300 pg/ml in the second half of their cycle. Anecdotal data indicates that levels over 90 to 100 pg/ml enable women to feel their best, maintain brain and cardiovascular health, and prevent bone loss (Vliet 1995).

Estrogen is also necessary for your body to utilize progesterone effectively. In fact, one of its functions is to create progesterone receptors. This is why many perimenopausal and menopausal women who faithfully apply progesterone cream daily don't see changes in their symptoms. When levels of estrogen are too low to create progesterone receptors, supplemental progesterone doesn't help. Recently a lot of research has focused on progesterone as an overlooked and critical hormone, but it's important to stress that progesterone doesn't do you any good if you don't have adequate estrogen.

By the time you're through perimenopause, you may have 20 percent of your estrogen left, but your progesterone levels will be near zero. As your ovaries don't produce hormones after menopause, your adrenal glands must take over production. Unfortunately, many women's adrenals are exhausted by years of continual stress or ill health and can't produce the levels of hormones necessary for them to feel good and function well.

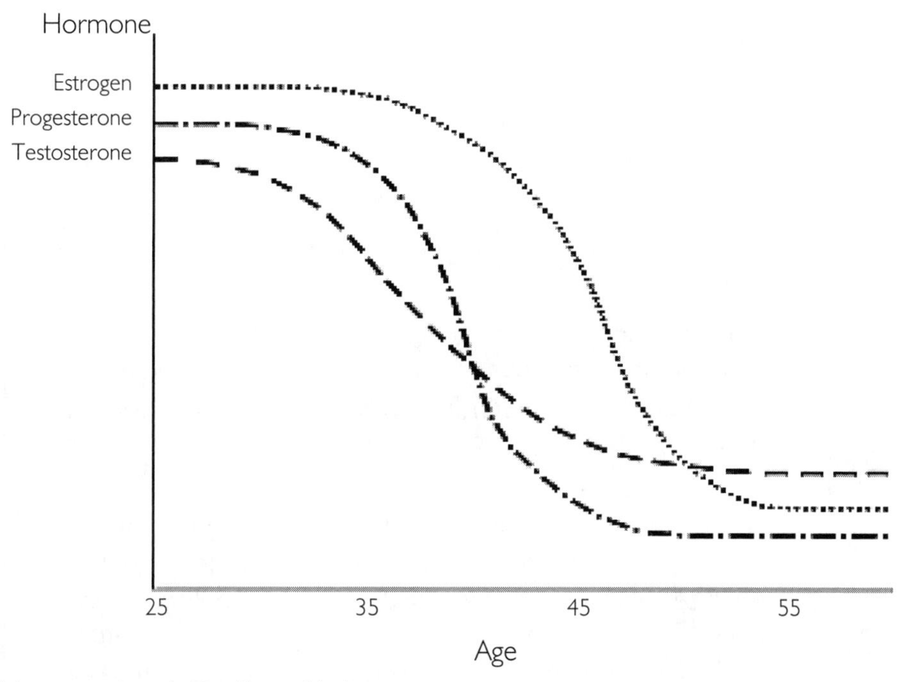

Hormone Levels Decline with Age

Most women don't know much about estrogen except that it's the hormone responsible for the development of female sex characteristics in adolescence and that it has a significant role in the menstrual cycle. Few women understand its profound effects on their bodies. In addition to regulating the menstrual cycle, estrogen affects, among other parts of the body, your heart and blood vessels, reproductive tract, urinary tract, bones, breasts, skin, hair, mucous membranes, pelvic muscles, and brain. The following table outlines some of the critical roles estrogen and progesterone play in the body.

	Estrogen's Effects on the Body	Progesterone's Effects on the Body
Memory and cognitive function	Important for short- and long-term memory and capacity for learning new associations (Sherwin 1996). Increases blood flow to the brain, improves cognition, and builds and maintains ner ve networks in the brain.	Critical in cognitive function and memory (Tanabe et al. 2004).
Bone	Slows bone loss (C. J. Gruber et al. 2002).	Stimulates new bone growth.
Breasts	Stimulates breast cells. Causes initial growth at puberty and maintains fullness.	Stops proliferation of cells in breasts. Protects against breast tenderness and pain and helps prevent breast cancer.
Weight	Causes weight gain around the hips and thighs when unbalanced by progesterone.	Balances estrogen to reduce middle-age weight gain around the hips and thighs.
Gallbladder	In excessive amounts and unbalanced by adequate progesterone, causes gallbladder problems (Chen and Huminer 1991).	Prevents gallbladder disease (Singletary, Van Thiel, and Eagon 1986).
Reproductive organs	Causes the endometrium to grow for conception. Regulates the menstrual cycle.	Maintains the endometrium, protects against excessive cell proliferation that can lead to reproductive cancers, is necessary for reproduction, and normalizes the menstrual cycle (Chen, Zhang, and Pollard 2003).

Heart and blood vessels	Alters thermoregulatory control of skin blood flow and relieves hot flashes and night sweats (Sherwin and Gelfand 1984). Protects against coronary artery disease (C. J. Gruber et al. 2002).	Protects the heart and maintains normal vascular tone and lipid profiles. Normalizes blood clotting and guards against strokes.
Nervous system	Responsible for nerve growth.	Important to nerve health and nerve regeneration.
Immune system	Key to optimal immune response.	Enhances immune function (Tanriverdi et al. 2003).
Sexual function	Necessary for sex drive and optimal functioning of genital organs.	Necessary for optimal sexual function.
Sleep	Necessary for the deep sleep phase of sleep, which is crucial to overall good health, especially muscle and nerve repair.	Necessary in the second half of the cycle to balance estrogen and promote regular sleep patterns.
Bladder/urinary function	Helps maintain vaginal and bladder tissues for sexual and bladder functions (Cardozo et al. 1998).	Prevents atrophy and dysfunction of the bladder.
Cell growth	Causes cell proliferation.	Balances excessive cell proliferation caused by estrogen.
Psychological functioning	Lower levels of estrogen have been tied to depression (Young et al. 2000).	Has a profound effect on mood (D. M. Gruber et al. 1999) and has a calming effect on brain neurons.
Relationships with other hormones	Important for optimum functioning of the thyroid but suppresses thyroid function when too high. Necessary to create progesterone receptors for optimal hormone balance.	Assists adrenal and thyroid function; maintains normal sensitivity of estrogen receptors; maintains optimal blood sugar levels; acts as a precursor of other hormones; modulates other hormones to ensure proper balance; balances estrogen.

EXERCISE: Assessing Symptoms of Deficient Estrogen

It's important to start with an inventory of your symptoms. They'll give you a good idea of what's going on in your body and if you have any imbalances. You may have several of these symptoms or just one. Check any of the following symptoms that you've experienced, whether currently or in the past:

- ☐ Back or leg pain
- ☐ Bladder problems
- ☐ Brain fog and memory problems
- ☐ Chronic colds and illness
- ☐ Constipation
- ☐ Decreased sex drive
- ☐ Deflated, sagging breasts
- ☐ Depression
- ☐ Dizziness
- ☐ Dry eyes
- ☐ Dry, thin skin
- ☐ Elevated cholesterol
- ☐ Excess hair growth
- ☐ Excessive fatigue
- ☐ Feeling bloated and swollen
- ☐ Feeling of bugs crawling on the skin
- ☐ Gum and tooth problems
- ☐ Hair loss
- ☐ Headaches
- ☐ Heart disease
- ☐ Heart palpitations
- ☐ Hot flashes
- ☐ Infertility
- ☐ Insomnia and sleep problems
- ☐ Irritability, mood swings, and weepiness
- ☐ Light or less frequent periods
- ☐ Looking older than your age
- ☐ Muscle and joint pain
- ☐ Osteoporosis or osteopenia
- ☐ Painful intercourse
- ☐ PMS
- ☐ Sinus problems
- ☐ Strange thoughts and psychological problems
- ☐ Tingling in the hands and feet
- ☐ Urinary incontinence or urgency
- ☐ Urinary tract infections
- ☐ Vaginal itching and pain
- ☐ Vision problems
- ☐ Voice changes
- ☐ Weight gain

In your journal, list all the of the symptoms you checked and use the format in the example below to note any additional information that will help your doctor understand what's going on, such as when in your cycle the different symptoms start or get worse. Do you have them throughout your cycle or just in the first or second half? Use a scale of 1 to 10 to rate severity, and describe how the symptom impacts your daily life.

Symptom	When It Occurs	Severity	How It Affects Your Daily Life
Incontinence	*Whenever I sneeze, laugh, or exercise.*	*7*	*I have to carry a change of underwear and clothes and wear a pad during exercise. It's embarrassing and stressful.*
Constipation	*It's been a problem for years.*	*8*	*I have to take laxatives every day, and I often feel tired and bloated.*

If you have only a minor symptom or two, such as water retention, this probably indicates only a slight deficiency of estrogen or excess of progesterone. The exact nature of the imbalance can be detected only through testing your estrogen and progesterone levels. What you and your doctor choose to do will be based on the severity of your symptoms and how much they affect your quality of life.

As you can see from the list of symptoms above, estrogen activity clearly isn't confined to your reproductive organs. It works throughout your entire body, affecting your overall health and ability to function. In recent years, extensive research on the effects of insufficient estrogen has revealed strong links to degenerative diseases like Alzheimer's and multiple sclerosis (Sandyk 1996). The medical community is finally waking up to the undeniable connections between changing hormone levels and illness and disease, and it's time for all of us to pay attention.

Your Brain and Estrogen

The effects of estrogen on brain function are particularly interesting. Women start out with fewer brain cells than men, but we have far more connections for each cell, which allows us to use several areas of our brain concurrently (which explains our ability to talk on the phone, cook dinner, and feed the baby at the same time!). Because we use a much larger portion of our brain than men, we need more energy and increased blood flow to fuel cognitive tasks (Witelson, Glezer, and Kigar 1995). One of the main functions of estrogen and thyroid hormones is to ensure optimum blood flow, so low estrogen or low thyroid results in less blood flow and therefore less brain function (Wise et al. 2002). So if you feel like you're losing your mind, maybe you just need to get your hormones back in balance!

Progesterone Levels Drop

Progesterone levels start to drop when you're in your thirties, and by your forties you're probably starting to have more and more cycles where you don't ovulate. If left unchecked, this can be the catalyst for unpleasant symptoms. Needless to say, waiting for perimenopausal symptoms to spur you into action isn't an effective way to manage hormone balance, because by the time you have symptoms, your estrogen and progesterone imbalance may be long-standing. Resulting problems, such as osteoporosis and heart disease, may have already begun to develop. Because you're still having periods during this time, you won't have obvious clues that you're not ovulating. The only way to get a handle on what's going on is to measure your estrogen and progesterone levels and test for ovulation.

Ovulating irregularly is the primary reason progesterone levels decrease before they should. If your progesterone is decreasing while you're still producing a relative abundance of estrogen, you should talk to your doctor about supplementing progesterone in anovulatory cycles. But there are several other reasons for decreased progesterone levels. Among the most common are high cortisol levels, environmental factors, and luteal phase defect.

High cortisol levels: Chronic stress, a poor diet, or lifestyle factors (not enough sleep, no exercise, and so on) can raise cortisol levels. Progesterone and cortisol compete for the same receptors in your body, so if your cortisol levels are too high for too long, progesterone can't reach its receptors and your body can't effectively utilize the progesterone it still has.

Environmental factors: Research over the last twenty years has revealed that progesterone levels have inexplicably started to drop at earlier and earlier ages—even affecting some women in their twenties or teens. There is convincing scientific evidence that environmental catalysts have hormone-disrupting effects, particularly exposure to certain synthetic chemicals in our everyday environment. These chemicals, which have only been around for about fifty years, are called *xenoestrogens* because they have estrogen-like structures and interfere with estrogen receptors. The resulting excessive estrogen exposure has been implicated in several health trends, including a dramatic increase in hormone-related cancers, a drop in sperm counts of 50 percent since 1940, and girls starting menstruation two years earlier, on average. This recent development should be taken seriously, particularly as so many children are now experiencing abnormal hormone problems (Moggs 2005).

Luteal phase defect: A common cause of infertility, this condition exists when ovulation occurs but a woman still doesn't produce adequate progesterone levels in the luteal phase, or second half of the cycle, so the uterus is never readied to receive an egg. Any of the following factors can cause luteal phase defect: premature loss of the corpus luteum (the egg sac that produces progesterone), inadequate follicle production, or failure of the uterine lining to respond to normal levels of progesterone.

EXERCISE: Assessing Symptoms of Deficient Progesterone

Here's a list of the side effects of inadequate progesterone with resulting excessive estrogen. Check any that apply to you, whether currently or in the past:

- ☐ Allergy symptoms
- ☐ Anxiety
- ☐ Bloating
- ☐ Brain fog and memory problems
- ☐ Breast tenderness
- ☐ Cervical dysplasia
- ☐ Cold hands and feet
- ☐ Decreased sex drive
- ☐ Depression
- ☐ Fat gain, especially around your hips and thighs
- ☐ Fibrocystic breasts
- ☐ Food cravings
- ☐ Gallbladder disease
- ☐ Hair loss
- ☐ Headaches
- ☐ Heartburn
- ☐ High blood pressure
- ☐ Hypoglycemia (diet-related mood and energy swings)
- ☐ Infertility
- ☐ Insomnia and sleep problems
- ☐ Irregular menstrual periods
- ☐ Irritability
- ☐ Looking older than your age
- ☐ Mood swings
- ☐ Osteoporosis or osteopenia
- ☐ PMS
- ☐ Thyroid dysfunction (see chapter 5 for symptoms)
- ☐ Uterine fibroids
- ☐ Water retention
- ☐ Weight gain

In your journal, list all of the symptoms you checked and use the format in the example below to note any additional information that will help your doctor understand what's going on, such as when in your cycle the different symptoms start or get worse. Do you have them throughout your cycle or just in the first or second half? Use a scale of 1 to 10 to rate severity, and describe how the symptom impacts your daily life.

Symptom	When It Occurs	Severity	How It Affects Your Daily Life
Headaches	*Almost every month—usually on day 1, but always during my period*	*9*	*I have a hard time functioning when I have a headache. It's very debilitating, and I usually have to lie down and rest.*
Breast tenderness	*Usually around ovulation*	*7*	*It's gotten so bad that I can't sleep on my stomach anymore.*

Testosterone

Testosterone is generally associated with men, just as estrogen is thought of as a female hormone. In recent years, however, research has shown that both of these hormones are important to both sexes. Although men produce twenty to thirty times more testosterone than women (Hertoghe 2006), this hormone also plays a key role in women's psychological and physical health, particularly in optimal sex drive, energy, and sense of well-being. When testosterone levels drop prior to menopause or following surgical or natural menopause, some women experience the symptoms listed below:

- Low energy or stamina
- Difficulty achieving orgasm
- Low sex drive
- Fatigue
- Poor muscle tone
- Increased body fat
- Heightened impatience or hostility
- Vaginal itching
- Accelerated bone loss
- Bladder incontinence
- Lack of coordination
- Decreased lean muscle mass

If you experience these symptoms, you should get your testosterone levels tested and evaluate whether a deficiency may be causing them. Research has shown that supplementing testosterone restores sex drive and function (Shifren et al. 2000).

On the other hand, testosterone levels in women can increase as estrogen levels decrease and get too high. Also, the lower levels of estrogen in perimenopause and menopause can allow existing testosterone to be more available and active and lead to the symptoms listed below:

- Hair growth, especially on the face and chest, in a male pattern
- Male-pattern baldness
- Deepening of the voice
- Increased muscle mass
- Redistribution of body fat
- Enlargement of the clitoris
- Acne
- Increased sweating

The best way to temper excessive testosterone is by replacing estrogen, which increases sex hormone binding protein, thus decreasing levels and availability of testosterone. (See chapter 8 for recommendations on replacing estrogen.)

TESTING OPTIONS

When you start a new diet, you're encouraged to write down everything you eat and when you eat it to help you see any patterns or problems in your eating habits. Likewise, monitoring and charting your hormone levels allows you to see how your hormones cycle and what your baseline levels are. This will help you understand and correct any imbalances that are revealed. The more precise your information is, the more effectively and quickly you'll be able to diagnose and treat your imbalances and start to feel better. It takes a little time to get a complete and accurate picture and really understand what's going on, but it's worth it.

Ovulation Self-Test

Though this test can't give you the detailed information you need to develop a treatment strategy, it will indicate whether you're experiencing anovulatory cycles and help you determine whether progesterone deficiency is an issue for you. Buy a reusable ovulation tester to find out whether you're ovulating each month. These testers are simple to use and involve testing your urine for a hormone indicative of ovulation. Another type of tester involves licking a supplied magnifying lens; when you subsequently look through the lens, it will show a distinctive pattern if you're ovulating. This technology is newer and not thought to be as accurate. But as it is reusable and much less expensive, you may want to try it and see whether it proves to be effective for you. Use the table below to log whether you ovulate in a given month and on what day of your cycle (*not* what day of the month). Another clue that you may have too little progesterone is if your menstrual cycle begins sooner than the normal twelve to fourteen days after ovulation.

Ovulation Dates					
January	February	March	April	May	June
July	August	September	October	November	December

Lab Tests

The following simple blood tests will give you and your doctor a clear picture of your hormone levels. It's always advisable to work with a hormone expert to evaluate and balance your hormones. If not ordered by a doctor, these tests will generally not be covered by your insurance. Doctors specializing in the hormone field generally understand how to apply effectively for insurance coverage for this testing, but even if your doctor orders the tests, some insurance companies may not cover them. Lab testing prices vary widely by geographical area and testing company.

Some lab companies offer hormone testing services without requiring a lab order from your doctor (see the Resources section for contact information). These tests may be less expensive than those offered through the lab recommended by your doctor, so you may want to get your testing done through one of these companies to save money.

If you're premenopausal, the tests described below should be done on the suggested days for the greatest accuracy and value in diagnosing potential imbalances. If you're postmenopausal, they may be done at any time. Tests should be done at about 8:00 A.M. on an empty stomach but having drunk two to three cups of water.

Progesterone: Measure progesterone levels between days nineteen and twenty-two of your menstrual cycle, when it's at its monthly peak, usually somewhere between 5 and 30 ng/ml (nanograms per milliliter). If this progesterone level is adequate (anything over 5 ng/ml shows you have ovulated) yet you still have symptoms of low progesterone, such as heavy periods and sore breasts, you should have your progesterone levels tested later in your cycle. This will tell you if the level is dropping off too rapidly because of a luteal phase defect.

Estrogen: Measure estrogen levels twice in the first month: first between days one and three to give you your lowest level of estrogen, and then between days nineteen and twenty-two (at the same time as you measure your progesterone level), when estrogen is high. If your cycle is irregular, you may have to test for more than one month to make sure you find the low and high points.

Testosterone: Testosterone may be measured at any time during your cycle, so if you're having other hormone levels tested, you can have your testosterone levels measured at the same time. It's a good idea to obtain a baseline reading of this hormone, as levels drop significantly at menopause and very low levels can cause unpleasant symptoms. (See the text box above for more information on potential symptoms.)

Follicle stimulating hormone: FSH levels should be tested between days nineteen and twenty-two of your cycle. This test measures the hormone that stimulates your ovaries to make more estrogen. The problem with this test is that when the ovaries start to slow down, estrogen production gets erratic, so levels of follicle stimulating hormone (FSH) may be high one month and low the next. However, it will tell you whether you're starting to run out of eggs and nearing menopause, so it is a useful indicator. An FSH test should never take the place of testing your estradiol levels, as the latter will tell you exactly how much estrogen your ovaries are producing.

Thyroid: Thyroid hormones will be explained more fully in chapter 5. Initial tests should be for levels of thyroid stimulating hormone (TSH), free T3, and free T4. These may be done at any time. Even if you're asymptomatic, these tests should be done to provide baseline levels.

Cortisol: Cortisol levels should be tested twice in one day at 8 a.m. (fasting) and 4 p.m., at any time in your cycle. See chapter 6 for full details.

Doctors have differing views on the best testing methodology. Most prefer blood tests because there's a huge body of long-term data to support results and ranges. Recently, some doctors have started to use saliva and twenty-four-hour urine testing as well, but many doctors feel these don't have as good a correlation to

Tests at a Glance

Here's a handy reference for what hormones you need to test when.

Type of Hormone	Day of Cycle to Measure and Times per Month
Progesterone	Once—between days 19 and 22 (additional testing may be needed)
Estradiol	Twice—between days 1 and 3 and between days 19 and 22
Testosterone	Once—anytime in your cycle
FSH	Once—between days 19 and 22
Thyroid (free T3, free T4, and TSH)	Once—anytime in your cycle (first thing in the morning is best)
Cortisol	Once—anytime in your cycle (two levels in one day, at 8 a.m. and 4 p.m.)

symptoms as blood tests do. The only saliva test that appears to be universally accepted is the salivary cortisol test, which is explained in chapter 6.

Have your doctor give you a copy of your lab results so you can copy the data into the table below, which has space for recording information for up to three tests of each hormone. This way you'll have a permanent record you can find easily for quick reference.

Lab Test Results				
Test	Date	Day of Cycle	Level	Reference Range from Lab Report
Progesterone				
Estradiol				
Testosterone				
FSH				
TSH				

Free T3				
Free T4				
Cortisol a.m.				
Cortisol p.m.				

RESTORING ESTROGEN AND PROGESTERONE BALANCE

It's important for all women, especially those in their perimenopausal years, to recognize patterns of imbalance between progesterone and estrogen. The information and exercises in this chapter have probably given you an idea of where you stand. The trick to good health and well-being during this period when estrogen and progesterone levels are shifting and changing is to restore their normal rhythms and balance, and chapter 8 covers this topic in detail. If you have plenty of estrogen left but it isn't adequately balanced with progesterone, the solution is to supplement progesterone in the last two weeks of the month to recreate a natural cycle. If, on the other hand, you're still ovulating but your estrogen levels have dropped significantly enough to cause you symptoms, you should consider supplementing estrogen either throughout the month or just when you experience low points, such as during days one through five.

The first thing to do is to have your hormone levels measured through lab tests. This will provide detailed information and alert you to any imbalances, such as subnormal estrogen or progesterone, or subnormal or elevated thyroid or cortisol. Even if these tests don't reflect declining hormone levels or imbalances, you should still track whether you ovulate every month for several months. This will let you know if you have a progesterone deficiency caused by lack of ovulation, and it's easier and cheaper than getting multiple lab tests.

Think about how your body is feeling. Notice when you experience different symptoms. Saying "I don't feel right" is the first step; the second is figuring out when and why you began to feel different; and the third and final step is doing something about it. Paying attention to your body and giving it the extra care needed to maintain hormone balance requires an investment of time and effort, and we all know that time is a valuable commodity. But don't cut corners when it comes to restoring your emotional and physical well-being. When you have the right amount of hormones and they're in balance, you'll feel great!

Things to Remember

- You lose up to 80 percent of your estrogen levels by menopause but almost all of your progesterone, so it's possible to still have too much unbalanced estrogen after menopause.
- You must have enough estrogen left in order for your body to be able to make progesterone receptors and utilize supplemental progesterone.
- Start to test for ovulation monthly, especially if you have any signs of excess estrogen.
- If you don't ovulate in a given month (and you still have some estrogen left), consider supplementing progesterone in the last two weeks of your cycle to balance estrogen levels.

CHAPTER 5

Out of Control: *Thyroid Imbalance*

Jeannie's Story

Jeannie, forty-two, is a mother of four. She always had enough energy for family, friends, community, and church, but as she approached forty her health began to change. It seemed that no matter what she ate, she gained weight. She put on sixty-five pounds in two years. Despite usually sleeping more than eight hours at night, she felt exhausted and began taking naps in the afternoon. She remembered that when she was in high school her mother began taking naps, so she figured this was just part of aging. Then her hair lost its shine and started falling out. Her skin became dry, and her feet scaly. Jeannie never wanted to do anything anymore. Even going out to dinner felt like an effort. Still, it didn't register that anything was wrong until her kids and husband started mentioning that she didn't seem like herself.

Jeannie scheduled an appointment with her doctor. Although she was afraid of what might be wrong, she was determined to find out what it was. When she told her symptoms to her doctor, he scheduled thyroid tests. When the results came back, she was distressed to learn that her thyroid hormone levels were significantly low, but she was also relieved to finally discover the cause of her problems. Jeannie's additional symptoms of heavy, shorter periods and sore breasts indicated she was no longer ovulating every month, leading to lower progesterone production and higher estrogen exposure, which could be causing further suppression of her thyroid.

Jeannie started on thyroid supplementation, and right away she started to lose weight and experience an improvement in many of her symptoms. Her doctor overlooked a significant issue though—he didn't suggest testing her progesterone levels to see if high estrogen and low progesterone were involved in her thyroid problems and if progesterone supplementation would have further supported and balanced her hormones. (Important lesson: Always ask for estrogen and progesterone tests as well as thyroid!)

METABOLISM AND YOUR THYROID

Advertisements about the many ways to improve metabolism bombard us from television, magazines, and the Internet. Diet books and supplement ads offer endless new approaches to increasing metabolism and triggering weight loss. But in actuality, your metabolic rate is set by your thyroid gland, so thyroid hormone is actually often the ideal natural weight-loss and energy-enhancing "supplement." It converts calories into energy, and it controls the rate at which cells and glands function and at which oxygen gets into cells. It helps the body effectively utilize energy and stay warm, and it's important for proper functioning of the brain, heart, muscles, and other organs. It also affects the chemistry of the brain and plays a key role in mental function, moods, and emotions.

The metabolic processes that control muscle maintenance and growth and fat burning are of particular significance for women. Thyroid malfunction is a major catalyst for the weight gain many of us experience as we age. With a sluggish thyroid, you can eat virtually nothing and still gain weight. When this is happening to you, advice from doctors, friends, and family to just eat less and exercise more is not only frustrating, it could prevent you from getting to the root of the problem. And if your thyroid condition goes untreated, you could end up with worse problems, such as depression, chronic fatigue, or fibromyalgia. Fibromyalgia, a disease that's becoming increasingly common among women, is characterized by widespread musculoskeletal pain, fatigue, and multiple tender points in localized areas, particularly the neck, spine, shoulders, and hips. It also can cause symptoms such as sleep disturbances, morning stiffness, irritable bowel syndrome, and anxiety.

What I Learned

I lived with thyroid malfunction for years and had most of the classic symptoms of low thyroid: chronic fatigue; cold, dry hands and feet; frequent colds and sinusitis; puffy skin; thin, ridged fingernails; and bouts of massive hair loss, which started after I had my last child at forty-one. I had no idea what was causing these symptoms, nor did I know that there might be a genetic connection. It wasn't until after I was diagnosed with MS and began researching hormones that I discovered a connection between low thyroid and MS (Karni and Abramsky 1999). Imagine my surprise when, in a conversation with my mother, I told her what I'd found, and she said, "Well, that makes sense. I've had to take thyroid medication since my midforties, and so have your grandmother and aunt." But since none of us had ever imagined that low thyroid could be related to a neurodegenerative condition like MS, this fact had never come up.

In one research study after another, I found that the thyroid is directly related to nerve health and repair (Fernandez et al. 2004). This illustrates why it's so important for you to include a complete family history in your hormone evaluation process. If I'd known about this genetic link, I would have looked more closely at the thyroid connection and would have been able to stop my downward spiral a lot sooner.

My doctor and I had tested my thyroid hormone levels as part of a thorough hormone evaluation when I discovered the link between hormones and my symptoms, but my tests were all in the "normal" range. My family medical history gave me the impetus I needed to go back to my doctor and say, "I know I have normal thyroid tests, but I just found out that all the women in my family have thyroid disease, and I'd like to try supplementing thyroid hormones." I was fortunate to have a good working relationship with an open-minded and creative doctor, so this new development convinced him to prescribe thyroid replacement for me. After trying several different thyroid therapies over the course of about six months, I found the optimum one, Armour Thyroid, which is a combination of both types of thyroid hormone, T3 and T4 (along with cortisol supplementation—more about that later), and my last remaining symptoms disappeared.

LOW THYROID: A VERY COMMON CONDITION

My experience was admittedly extreme, with exaggerated and debilitating symptoms. But research shows that almost *eight million* American women have thyroid disease (Staub et al. 1992) and many more go undiagnosed. Worldwide estimates of numbers of people with thyroid problems are rising steadily. Thyroid expert and researcher Dr. Broda Barnes estimated that 30 percent of people had hypothyroidism, and noted endocrinologist Dr. Jacques Hertoghe suggested that it could be as high as 80 percent (Durrant-Peatfield 2002). It's sobering to realize that this imbalance, which affects almost every aspect of health, is frequently misdiagnosed, misunderstood, and overlooked.

This is why, if you have symptoms of low thyroid function, it is so important to test and treat the symptoms without delay. Your thyroid gland controls the production of energy for every bodily activity. It is critical to appetite, sex drive, sleep, and psychological well-being. So what does low thyroid leave you with? An unhappy, tired, irritable, overweight woman who isn't interested in sex . . . sound familiar?

HOW YOUR THYROID WORKS

To work effectively with your doctor to see how well your thyroid is functioning, you need to have a general understanding of how the thyroid works. Here are the basics: Your thyroid gland is regulated by your pituitary gland, a small endocrine gland attached to the base of your brain. Your pituitary gland produces thyroid stimulating hormone (TSH), which stimulates your thyroid gland to produce two key hormones—T3 (triiodothyronine) and T4 (thyroxine)—in response to your body's needs. T4 blood levels are higher than T3, but T3 is far more potent and biologically active. The body converts T4 to T3 as needed. Your pituitary gland is, in turn, regulated by your hypothalamus, a small part of your brain just above it. The hypothalamus produces thyrotropin releasing hormone (TRH), which stimulates the pituitary gland to release TSH.

Your thyroid can malfunction in one of two ways: It can become either underactive (hypothyroidism) or overactive (hyperthyroidism). When your T3 and T4 levels drop too low, your pituitary gland, located in your brain, produces thyroid stimulating hormone, which does exactly what its name indicates—it stimulates your thyroid to produce more T3 and T4. Increasing TSH levels are a sign that thyroid hormone levels are dropping and that you should be on the lookout for symptoms of low thyroid.

There have been many recent advancements in understanding the thyroid in general, and thyroid testing specifically. But unfortunately, with their busy schedules, doctors often have little time to keep up with ongoing research. So you'll have to be knowledgeable when you bring this topic up for discussion.

Hypothyroidism

Hypothyroidism occurs when your thyroid doesn't make enough thyroid hormones to meet the needs of your body. The reasons are varied and include genetic inheritance, exposure to certain viruses, an iodine deficiency, direct physical trauma to the thyroid, indirect trauma (such as whiplash), autoimmune disease, environmental toxins, or thyroid antibodies. Thyroid antibodies are produced in response to your body's mistaken belief that it is being attacked. When faced with a perceived foreign threat, the immune system produces antibodies to attack and disarm the threat. Unfortunately, antibodies are sometimes produced in response to the body's own tissues and substances, including thyroid hormones, and this immune response can impair thyroid function. If thyroid antibodies are the root cause, it usually takes your body a long time, sometimes many years, to reach full-blown hypothyroidism. You'll most likely see symptoms gradually creep up year by year, but since the symptoms so closely mimic the aging process, people often interpret them as simply signs of getting older.

Hypothyroidism can occur not only as a result of undersecretion of thyroid hormone from the thyroid gland, which is called *primary hypothyroidism*, but also as a result of damage to, or disease of, the pituitary or hypothalamus, called *central hypothyroidism*. Two other terms are often applied to central hypothyroidism, which is often found in chronically ill patients: *secondary hypothyroidism* in the case of pituitary disease, or *tertiary hypothyroidism* in the case of hypothalamic dysfunction. Both of these conditions involve a reduction in circulating thyroid hormones as a result of inadequate stimulation of the thyroid gland by TSH (Miller 1998).

As you can see, hypothyroidism is a complex condition, and to confuse us and our doctors further, many women have *functional hypothyroidism*. This means that you have symptoms of low thyroid even though all your thyroid tests are normal. You may have slightly increased levels of TSH, but not enough to be considered hypothyroid. What most women (and many times their doctors as well) don't realize is that a "normal" range for thyroid lab tests is just a guideline; many women may require higher (or lower) levels to be healthy and feel well. Lab results must be evaluated along with your entire clinical picture to be meaningful.

Hypothyroidism is a very common condition in perimenopause, when estrogen and progesterone levels become imbalanced. Unbalanced estrogen is one of the primary causes because, as you may recall, when the estrogen-to-progesterone ratio goes up, thyroid hormone levels go down. Balancing estrogen with progesterone is often the key to rebalancing your thyroid and returning your levels of thyroid hormones to normal. Another common cause of hypothyroidism relates to the fact that your ovaries have thyroid hormone receptors (and your thyroid has ovarian hormone receptors). So when your ovaries slow drastically at menopause, thyroid function is also often affected.

The Iodine Connection

Lack of iodine, the main cause of hypothyroidism in developing countries, results in impaired thyroid hormone synthesis. Many people in the United States believe that iodine deficiency no longer exists in this country as it does in developing countries, but that's not the case. The most recent National Health and Nutrition Examination Survey (with data gathered between 1988 and 1994) showed that the average U.S. daily dietary iodine intake has fallen from 320 mcg (micrograms) to 145 mcg over the past twenty years. Iodine deficiency was found in 14.9 percent of adult women, a 4.5-fold increase over the iodine deficiency found in the previous survey, done from 1971 through 1974 (Hollowell et al. 1998).

Iodide is added to table salt, but in very small amounts, and many people are trying to restrict their salt intake because of the connection between salt and hypertension. In the past, adequate levels of iodine could be obtained from vegetables grown in iodine-rich soil, but aggressive farming practices have depleted our soil of many minerals, including iodine, resulting in iodine-poor produce. Much higher amounts of iodine were added to bread and milk until the 1980s to compensate for iodine-depleted soil, but that practice was stopped and the amount of iodine added to salt continues to shrink. Iodized salt contains only 74 mcg of iodine per gram of salt, which isn't enough to meet iodine requirements for the human body—it's simply a minimum level designed to prevent goiter and cretinism. The recommended daily allowance (RDA) for iodine is 150 mcg, but recent research suggests this is too low to allow the body to make sufficient thyroid hormones, and higher levels of supplementation may be required by the body for optimum health (Abraham, Flechas, and Hakala 2002b). Iodine is utilized by every hormone receptor in the body, so deficient iodine can result in widespread hormonal imbalances, causing problems such as ovarian cysts, thyroid goiter, and thyroid adenomas.

Another sign of low iodine is fibrocystic breast disease (Ghent et al. 1993), characterized by lumpy, sore, cystic breasts. To avoid this condition, research shows that you should get at least 5 milligrams of iodine per day (Abraham, Flechas, and Hakala 2002a). But to get this much iodine from iodized salt, you'd have to consume a whopping (and life-threatening) 68 grams of salt. Given the problems with excessive salt consumption, it's clearly better to get your iodine from a supplement. The Japanese population, which has the lowest rate of cancers of the breast and the female reproductive system, consumes approximately 13.8 milligrams (13,800 mcg) of iodine per day, mostly from sea vegetables. If you have fibrocystic breast disease, you may have an increased risk of breast cancer (Vorherr 1986) and should consider taking the iodine loading test explained in the "Lab Tests for Thyroid Function" section below to determine if you have an iodine deficiency.

EXERCISE: Assessing Symptoms of Hypothyroidism

Study the list of low thyroid symptoms below and check any that apply to you:

- ☐ Anxiety
- ☐ Asthma
- ☐ Attention-deficit/hyperactivity disorder
- ☐ Back or leg pain
- ☐ Bladder irritation
- ☐ Bluish skin, nail beds, lips, or mucous membranes
- ☐ Bowel problems
- ☐ Brain fog and memory problems
- ☐ Breathlessness
- ☐ Brittle, thin, ridged fingernails
- ☐ Carpal tunnel syndrome
- ☐ Cervical dysplasia
- ☐ Chronic colds and illness
- ☐ Chronic constipation
- ☐ Cold hands and feet
- ☐ Deafness or hearing problems
- ☐ Decreased sex drive
- ☐ Depression
- ☐ Dry, coarse skin
- ☐ Early menopause
- ☐ Easy bruising
- ☐ Eczema and psoriasis
- ☐ Elevated cholesterol
- ☐ Enlarged abdomen
- ☐ Excessive fatigue
- ☐ Fibrocystic breast disease
- ☐ Fibromyalgia

- ☐ Flatulence
- ☐ Food cravings
- ☐ Hair loss
- ☐ Halitosis
- ☐ Headaches
- ☐ Heart enlargement
- ☐ Heart palpitations
- ☐ Hemorrhoids
- ☐ High blood pressure
- ☐ Hoarse voice
- ☐ Infertility
- ☐ Insomnia and sleep problems
- ☐ Intolerance of cold or heat
- ☐ Lack of sweating
- ☐ Listless, dull eyes
- ☐ Liver pain or swelling
- ☐ Looking older than your age
- ☐ Loss of body hair
- ☐ Low basal body temperature
- ☐ Low blood pressure
- ☐ Muscle weakness
- ☐ Pain in the hands and feet
- ☐ Painful or irregular periods
- ☐ Pale lips
- ☐ Pale or yellow skin
- ☐ PMS
- ☐ Puffy face and eyelids
- ☐ Recurrent upper respiratory and urinary infections
- ☐ Restless legs syndrome
- ☐ Scalloped, thick, or wasting tongue
- ☐ Slow speech
- ☐ Slowed Achilles reflex
- ☐ Sluggish movement
- ☐ Stiffness and pain
- ☐ Strange thoughts and psychological problems
- ☐ Swollen legs and feet
- ☐ Thickening of the neck or goiter
- ☐ Thinning, dry, coarse, brittle hair
- ☐ Thinning eyebrows, especially at the outer ends
- ☐ Tingling in the hands and feet
- ☐ Tinnitus
- ☐ Urinary urgency and frequency
- ☐ Vision problems
- ☐ Voice changes
- ☐ Weak, slow, or soft pulse
- ☐ Weight gain
- ☐ Yeast infections
- ☐ Yellowish skin or whites of the eyes

In your journal, write down all of the symptoms you checked, using the format in the example below. Note any details, such as when you first got the symptom, how long you've had it, and whether it's getting worse or better. Can you remember any trigger or event that may have precipitated the symptom, such as pregnancy or an accident or injury?

Symptom	When It Began	Getting Worse or Better?
My periods are getting closer together. I have one every 2 to 3 weeks.	*Age 40*	*Worse*
Hair loss: The hair on my head is getting thin and my eyebrows are very sparse.	*After my last child was born, when I was 38*	*Worse*

TESTING YOUR THYROID FUNCTION

If you have several of the symptoms above, or one or two serious or uncomfortable ones, schedule an appointment with your doctor as soon as possible to review them and arrange for a thorough thyroid evaluation, including the tests listed below, under "Lab Tests for Thyroid Function." If your symptoms turn out to be unrelated to low thyroid, they may be caused by poor physical conditioning, cortisol deficiency, vitamin or mineral deficiencies (particularly of folic acid, B_{12}, and B_1), use of beta-blocking drugs, very low calorie intake, iodine deficiency, or thyroid hormone resistance (Honeyman-Lowe and Lowe 2003). You and your doctor should evaluate these other potential causes.

Self-Tests for Thyroid Function

If you're concerned about your thyroid function but must wait for a doctor's appointment to get your levels tested, there are a couple of simple and inexpensive home tests you can do to investigate the situation in the meanwhile.

IODINE DEFICIENCY TEST

You can do this easy and inexpensive test at home to determine if iodine deficiency might be the cause of your thyroid problem. If you use little salt, or noniodized salt, you may be deficient, and iodine is essential for the thyroid gland to produce T4.

Buy a 2 percent tincture of iodine at the drugstore. With the applicator or a cotton swab, dab a patch of iodine the size of a silver dollar (about one inch across) on your stomach or thigh. If your iodine level is normal, the spot will still be there after twenty-four hours. If it disappears in less than twenty-four hours, you're iodine deficient. The faster it disappears, the greater your deficiency. Without sufficient iodine, you'll have low thyroid activity and lessened ability to convert T4 to T3. This explains why many people don't respond to thyroid supplementation.

If your iodine spot disappears quickly, review carefully the list of hypothyroid symptoms earlier in this chapter. If you have several of them, or one or two serious ones, contact your doctor and set up an appointment for a thyroid check and testing.

SWALLOW TEST

This quick and easy self-exam can be used to help detect an enlarged thyroid gland. This is important information, as it indicates thyroid malfunction and the need for further testing. All you need is a glass of water and a mirror, and to know exactly where your thyroid gland is located: It's at the base of the front of your neck, between your Adam's apple and your collarbone. While looking at this area in the mirror, tip your head back and take a drink of water. As you swallow, note any bulging or protrusion in the thyroid area (don't be distracted by your Adam's apple, which is located above the thyroid). If you're at all uncertain, repeat the process until you're sure whether or not you see a bulge. If you notice any bulges, you may have a thyroid problem, in which case you should consult with your doctor and arrange for the lab tests described below as soon as possible.

BASAL BODY TEMPERATURE TEST FOR HYPOTHYROIDISM

This basal body temperature test measures the most basic function of the thyroid gland: its ability to regulate body temperature. Try this test if you suspect that your thyroid isn't functioning at its best or if your laboratory results are normal but you still have many bothersome symptoms of low thyroid. If your temperature is below 97.8°F, this evidence of low thyroid or low metabolic function may convince your doctor to give you a trial course of thyroid hormone replacement.

Many doctors who have successfully used this method to diagnose low thyroid recommend that you do this simple test for ten days in a row starting on day 1 of your cycle. If you still have a period, begin on day one of your period; if not, you can do it anytime. The night before testing, shake down a glass basal thermometer to below 95°F. The next morning, as soon as you wake up and before you get out of bed, put the thermometer under your arm with the bulb in your armpit, next to your skin. Lie still for ten minutes. Remove the thermometer, read it, and record the result below. A normal reading falls between 97.8°F and 98.2°F. If yours is below this range, you probably have hypothyroidism. If it's higher, you may have hyperthyroidism (or a low-grade infection).

Basal Body Temperature										
Day of cycle	1	2	3	4	5	6	7	8	9	10
Date										
Temperature										

In your journal, jot down anything that might have affected your temperature. For instance, if you forgot to take your temperature one day, or got up to go to the bathroom before testing on another day, that could have caused an artificially higher reading. Are your readings consistently below 97.8°F? If so, you should make an appointment to have your thyroid function tested and evaluated.

Lab Tests for Thyroid Function

If self-tests indicate that you may have problems with your thyroid function, it's important that you undergo lab tests to see exactly what's going on. However, you may face some resistance from your doctor, so you must be well-informed and persistent. This is especially important if weight gain is one of your primary symptoms (as it is for many women). When you ask your doctor what's causing your weight gain, chances are you'll get sympathy, a lecture, or a prescription:

Sympathy: "You're trying to do too much. You just need to slow down and rest; sometimes women eat too much when they're stressed."

Lecture: "You obviously need to cut back on what you eat. Cut out the sweets (or carbohydrates or meat or fats) and exercise more!"

Prescription: Your doctor will probably recommend diet pills or antidepressants, not hormone therapy.

If you're eating sensibly (or hardly at all) and are active, you shouldn't have a problem with weight gain. Getting any of the above responses is bound to frustrate you, so if this happens, use your frustration productively. This is not the time to be passive; this is your health we're talking about. Take a deep breath and calmly request the lab tests listed below for thyroid function. It's worth it to find out if low thyroid, not too many calories or lack of exercise, is causing your symptoms. In addition to testing levels of various thyroid hormones, it's also important to check levels of estrogen and progesterone, as progesterone deficiency can suppress your thyroid function. I know from my own experience, the experiences of my friends, and years of research that many women with low thyroid function suffer needlessly. With the right hormone therapy, these same women are restored to full energy and health. With education and persistence you can get to the root of the problem.

TSH, T3, AND T4 TESTS

The first step in evaluating thyroid function is to measure your levels of thyroid stimulating hormone. In early hypothyroidism, TSH levels rise to stimulate production of thyroid hormones. At this point, your T3 and T4 levels may still be relatively normal, but as the malfunction progresses, TSH keeps rising and levels of T3 and T4 drop further. Unfortunately, if your TSH, T3, and T4 are still in the low normal range, most doctors are reluctant to treat you, even when you have profound symptoms of hypothyroidism. Another problem is that thyroid testing is notoriously inaccurate because hormone levels are individual to each woman; what may be a normal and completely adequate level for one may be too low for another.

If you have central hypothyroidism caused by damage to or disease of the pituitary or hypothalamus, you'll have signs and symptoms of hypothyroidism, but it will be difficult for anyone other than a trained thyroid specialist to interpret your lab results. With secondary hypothyroidism, the general pattern is that TSH levels are normal or low, T4 is reduced, and T3 is normal or reduced (Hueston 2001). The confusion comes in because even if your TSH levels are normal, only a small portion of your TSH molecules are functioning normally, resulting in inadequate thyroid function (Miller 1998). Therefore, a doctor who isn't trained in this specialty will generally interpret these results to mean that you don't have a thyroid problem. This is another reason why it is so important that symptoms be the critical factor in deciding whether thyroid supplementation might be worthwhile. This problem with interpreting TSH levels also makes managing central hypothyroidism more complicated because TSH can't be used to monitor response to replacement therapy as it is in primary hypothyroidism. Nevertheless, thyroid replacement can lead to profound improvements, especially if the person suffers from a chronic disease.

Despite the shortcomings of thyroid testing, getting your levels tested is important for several reasons. First, it's still the best way to diagnose primary hypothyroidism. Second, even if your symptoms are caused by some other hormone imbalance, having these baseline levels will help you identify potential problems if your levels change in the future. Your initial tests should include TSH, free T4, and free T3. More and more doctors are recommending you test these *free* levels, meaning the amount of hormone that's actually biologically active in your body—rather than *total* levels.

TSH levels have been the center of controversy for a long time. Many doctors adhere rigidly to the "normal" ranges set out and won't treat anyone whose thyroid hormones fall within this range. In January 2003, the American Association of Clinical Endocrinologists finally recognized that the range of 0.3 to 5 was far too broad and recommended that doctors "consider treatment for patients who test outside a . . . target TSH level of 0.3 to 3.0" (American Association of Clinical Endocrinologists 2003). If you were tested before 2003, you may have fallen within the previously higher "normal" range, so may have been told your thyroid function was fine. Many doctors who work routinely with thyroid problems now treat women whose TSH levels are much lower, such as over 2.0 or 2.5. It's also important to compare lab results over time; for instance, if your TSH was 0.4 last year and 1.8 this year—both normal, but rising with time—this indicates that some sort of change is occurring that should be watched closely.

OTHER THYROID LAB TESTS

If your TSH level is normal but you have a family history of thyroid disease, autoimmune disease, or persistent thyroid symptoms, consider testing for thyroid antibodies as well, specifically thyroid peroxidase antibodies (TPOab), thyroglobulin antibodies (TgAb), and thyrotropin receptor antibodies (TRAb). There are two other thyroid lab tests you or your doctor may consider: reverse T3 and an iodine loading test.

Reverse T3: This test allows you to see if excess reverse T3 might be causing your thyroid symptoms. The thyroid produces T4, most of which is converted into T3 outside the thyroid gland. However, some T4 is converted into reverse T3 (RT3), which is produced as a way to help clear T4 from the body. At the same time, RT3 also binds with and blocks the action of T3. Excessive dieting, illness, or excess cortisol output due to stress can all inhibit the conversion of T4 to T3 and increase the conversion of T4 to RT3. This slows the body's metabolism and thereby slows elimination of reverse T3 from the body, leading to increased levels.

Iodine loading test: In this twenty-four-hour urine test, you ingest 50 mg of iodine and then collect all your urine over the next twenty-four hours. The premise is that if you have enough iodine, most of the 50 mg of iodine will be excreted in your urine over the twenty-four-hour period. If you're iodine deficient, you'll retain more of the supplemental iodine, so a smaller amount will be in your urine. If the amount of iodine measured is less than 90 percent, you're presumed to be iodine deficient.

Lauren's Story

Lauren was only thirty-four when she began to feel increasingly tired and confused and started having trouble concentrating. She hadn't changed her diet, she was sleeping well, and she wasn't under any more stress than normal, yet she had trouble finishing projects at work and had to go over things again and again to make sense of them. She had difficulty handling her kids' schedules and was late to or missed many of their activities. Things came to a head when she arrived late at her daughter's school play, burst into tears when she couldn't find a parking space, then fell asleep during the play. When she woke with a start during the applause and saw her daughter glaring at her, she finally realized that something wasn't right.

But when she started getting physical symptoms, she realized something was seriously wrong: Her thinning hair and dry skin were hard enough to deal with, but the day the young man behind the deli counter congratulated her on her "pregnancy," she was forced into action. Fortunately, her doctor recognized her symptoms immediately and diagnosed hypothyroidism. Lauren started on a prescription for combination T4 and T3 therapy. This eased her symptoms, and her daughter even mentioned how different she seemed.

TREATING HYPOTHYROIDISM

The good news about hypothyroidism is that it's easy to treat, and even better news is that treatment has the potential to make you feel better very quickly. The bad news is that therapy for mild hypothyroidism is still controversial in the medical community, which is why it's extremely important that you have a good understanding of thyroid dysfunction. If your blood tests don't show very high levels of TSH and/or very low levels of T3 and T4, your doctor may be reluctant to prescribe thyroid hormone replacement. This is even more of a problem if you're subclinical and your tests don't show any deficiency. However, if your symptoms are clearly indicative of low thyroid, most doctors experienced in working with thyroid disorders will generally agree to a trial of low-dose thyroid supplementation. In this case, it's important to continue to monitor your levels closely to make sure you don't end up with *hyper*thyroidism. If you have more significant indicators of thyroid dysfunction, such as goiter, thyroid antibodies, manic-depressive disorder, fertility problems, or a family history of thyroid problems, your doctor will also probably agree to try thyroid treatment even if your tests are normal.

In either of these situations, your doctor may request you to sign a waiver stating that you've requested this therapy even though your tests fall within "normal" limits. In these litigious times, this is standard operating procedure. It's also a reasonable request, because without confirming lab results, this falls outside of *standard-of-care* treatment, which in legal terms means "the level at which the average, prudent provider in a given community would practice. It is how similarly qualified practitioners would have managed the patient's care under the same or similar circumstances" (MedicineNet 2006). This guideline is used in determining liability in medical malpractice cases. Doctors who aren't following the standard of care have more liability, and if we want our doctors to partner with us, we have to understand and respect their responsibilities and assume ours. If your doctor isn't comfortable working with you to find a solution, it's time to find another doctor or to ask for a referral to an endocrinologist—a doctor who specializes in hormones.

Treatment alternatives for hypothyroidism can be confusing. Your doctor will most likely want you to try T4 therapy first, as this is the current standard of care. While some do well on this therapy, recent research has shown that many women have difficulty converting T4 to T3 because of stress, diet, illness, or more esoteric biochemical issues, and to be effective, T4 must be converted to T3. Some estimates suggest that up to 50 percent of women have a better experience with a replacement therapy that includes T3. Clinical study results have also supported this (Bunevicius et al. 1999), adding further credence to what many women are reporting to their doctors: that they do better when they use both T3 and T4.

One of the pioneers of thyroid research and treatment was Dr. Broda Barnes, who treated thousands of hypothyroid patients in the 1960s and 1970s. He recommended starting doses of Armour Thyroid (a T3/T4 combination product derived from pigs) as follows: Children over six could start at one-half grain (one grain is a 60 mg pill), teenagers and adults at one grain, and very large men or women at two grains. He noted that changes in symptoms generally occurred within the first month or two. If patients started to feel better but all symptoms didn't resolve after two months, he suggested the dose be reevaluated and recommended that teenagers increase their dose by one-half grain and adults by one grain. He suggested this process be repeated until all symptoms were resolved at the lowest possible dose. He found that this dose was most commonly two grains in his adult patients—with fewer requiring three and rarely four (Barnes and Galton 1976).

Unfortunately, trial and error is the only way to arrive at the dose that's right for you, and you have to be the best judge of what that is. Bear in mind that feelings of well-being and symptom resolution may fade after a couple of days or a week. If this happens, don't panic—it usually just means that the dose is too low (or that you also have adrenal fatigue, which is explained at the end of this chapter). Once your body adjusts, it wants more, and this signals that it's time to increase your dose. Your doctor will be instrumental in guiding you through this process.

T4 treatment: Most doctors still prescribe a replacement drug consisting solely of T4, such as Synthroid, Levothroid, or Levoxyl (all brand names for levothyroxine), which are some of the most commonly prescribed medications in the United States today. Dosing is generally 1 microgram per pound of body weight, so if you weigh 100 pounds, you would probably take 100 mcg of T4. But your doctor will probably start you at a lower dose and raise it slowly to find your optimal dose, starting you at 25 to 50 mcg and going up by 25 mcg every week until your symptoms resolve. If your doctor wants you to start with T4 treatment but you don't get total resolution, ask to try a combination T3 and T4 product.

T3 and T4 combination treatment: Many doctors, noticing that their patients don't get complete relief on T4 alone, have been adding T3 to their therapy. T4 (such as Synthroid) can be taken in conjunction with T3 (such as Cytomel, or liothyronine). Other products with a combination of T3 and T4 are desiccated thyroid (Armour or generics), made from dried pig or cow thyroid, and Thyrolar (liotrix), a combination of synthetic T4 and T3.

T3 treatment: Exciting new research suggests that higher-dose T3 therapy alone may be successful in treating specific diseases such as fibromyalgia and chronic fatigue syndrome. It's possible that these diseases are symptoms of peripheral thyroid resistance, a condition that responds to slowly increasing doses of T3 (Lowe 2000).

Finding the optimal dose of thyroid hormones may involve trying a couple of different dosing schedules, and this may take several months. This is another reason why it's important to find a doctor you're comfortable with; you need someone to support you through this sometimes frustrating process. You may be lucky and find the right dose immediately, but even if it takes time, the result is worth it!

Before you start on thyroid replacement, you should always check levels of estrogen and progesterone to see if deficient progesterone could be the cause of suppressed thyroid function. When this is the case, you simply need to supplement progesterone in the last two weeks of your cycle to balance estrogen and thereby normalize your thyroid function, an approach that would have made a big difference for Sara.

Sara's Story

Sara is a thirty-seven-year-old who started to experience excessive menstrual bleeding at thirty-five. Her ob-gyn was unaware that estrogen and progesterone imbalance might be the cause of her problem, so he resorted to recommending the only solution he knew—a hysterectomy. Holistically oriented, Sara didn't want to have a hysterectomy. But after a year and a half of living with anxiety over unpredictable flooding and the embarrassment of bleeding through her clothes on several occasions, she didn't feel she had any alternatives.

Sara's doctor put her on oral estrogen replacement after her surgery because of her age. Sticking to the common practice following a hysterectomy, her doctor didn't prescribe progesterone supplementation since she no longer had a uterus. (The standard-of-care approach is to only use progesterone to counteract cell proliferation in the uterus.) Within three months Sara had become so tired that she had a hard time getting through the workday. Her hair began to fall out, and she gained weight even though she hadn't changed her eating habits. She felt certain that these symptoms were related to her hysterectomy even though her doctor said they weren't. Sensing that something was wrong with her hormones, she asked him to test her hormone levels. Because of her fatigue and weight gain symptoms, he only tested her thyroid hormone levels. When they came back at the low end of the normal range, her doctor told her again that her symptoms weren't related to the surgery.

Neither Sara nor her doctor understood that she was experiencing functional hypothyroidism brought on by replacing only estrogen. Even though she no longer had her uterus, she still had estrogen- and progesterone-sensitive tissues throughout her body that needed progesterone—her brain, nervous system, and heart, to name a few! The unchallenged estrogen had the effect of suppressing Sara's thyroid, causing all the unpleasant symptoms associated with low thyroid function. Adding progesterone would have balanced the estrogen and returned her thyroid function to normal.

HYPERTHYROIDISM

Hyperthyroidism is the opposite of hypothyroidism. Instead of producing too little thyroid hormone, in hyperthyroidism your thyroid becomes overactive and produces too much. The most common form is Graves' disease, and even it isn't very common, affecting only about 2 percent of women, mostly during their thirties and forties (Reid and Wheeler 2005). On the surface, hyperthyroidism may sound attractive. After all, too little thyroid means weight gain and exhaustion, so too much should mean svelte and lively, right? Unfortunately, too much of a good thing generally turns out to be a bad thing, and in this case, too much thyroid hormone can damage your cells, particularly in your heart and muscles. It can also increase your risk of osteoporosis.

With hyperthyroidism, the body's metabolism increases. You feel hotter than those around you and continue to lose weight even though you may be eating more. (However, some people with hyperthyroidism actually gain weight due to increased appetite.) It's also common to be very tired at the end of the day, but then be wired, agitated, and unable to sleep. Your hands may tremble, you may be irritable, and you may have heart palpitations. You'll usually find yourself becoming easily upset. When hyperthyroidism is severe, you can suffer shortness of breath, chest pain, and muscle weakness. Usually the symptoms of hyperthyroidism are so gradual in their onset that you don't realize what's happening at first. Your symptoms may continue for weeks or months before you realize you have a problem.

EXERCISE: Assessing Symptoms of Hyperthyroidism

The symptoms listed below are associated with hyperthyroidism. Check any that apply to you:

- ☐ Anxiety
- ☐ Breathlessness
- ☐ Coarsening and reddening of the skin on your shins
- ☐ Excessive fatigue
- ☐ Fast heart rate
- ☐ Hair loss
- ☐ Heart palpitations
- ☐ Heat intolerance
- ☐ Increased bowel movements or diarrhea
- ☐ Insomnia and sleep problems
- ☐ Light or absent menstrual periods
- ☐ Muscle weakness
- ☐ Nervousness
- ☐ Protruding eyes
- ☐ Staring gaze
- ☐ Thickening of the neck or goiter
- ☐ Trembling hands
- ☐ Warm, moist skin
- ☐ Weight loss

In your journal, write down all of the symptoms you checked, using the format in the example below. Note any details, such as when you first got the symptom, how long you've had it, and whether it's getting worse or better.

Symptom	**When It Began**	**Getting Worse or Better?**
Heart palpitations	*It started in 1999, when I was pregnant.*	*Worse*
Protruding eyes	*Started in 2002.*	*Worse*

If you have several of the symptoms, or one or two serious or uncomfortable ones, schedule an appointment with your doctor as soon as possible to review them and arrange for a thorough thyroid evaluation and the tests listed in the "Lab Tests for Thyroid Function" section above.

TREATING HYPERTHYROIDISM

There are several treatments for hyperthyroidism. The first is to do nothing and just wait and see, because mild forms of hyperthyroidism sometimes resolve without intervention. If symptoms become bothersome, one option is to treat the symptoms of anxiety and nervousness with medication, such as the muscle relaxant Valium (diazepam) and/or beta-blockers.

When the condition is more serious and symptoms more severe, antithyroid medication can be used to slow down hormone production. In severe cases, the more extreme choice of treatment is *thyroid ablation*, which effectively destroys much, or all, of your thyroid with radioactive iodine or surgery. Unfortunately, these treatments often replace one problem with another, resulting in hypothyroidism that then must be treated with thyroid hormone replacement.

Finally, as in hypothyroidism, you may have *subclinical* hyperthyroidism—symptoms of hyperthyroidism but normal test results. The results will likely show low TSH and normal T3 and T4. Tests to diagnose hyperthyroidism are the same as those for hypothyroidism: TSH, T3, and T4. If the first three tests are normal but your symptoms persist, you should also do thyroid antibody tests to see if antibodies could be the root cause of your problem.

RESTORING THYROID BALANCE

There's no escaping that our hormones are interrelated. Thyroid hormones have a mutually dependent relationship with estrogen and progesterone: Your ovaries have thyroid hormone receptors, and your thyroid has receptors for estrogen and progesterone. When one hormone is deficient or out of balance, the others don't work well either. Low thyroid is one of the most common causes of menstrual problems, lower estrogen and progesterone production, and infertility.

Your adrenal glands are also inextricably linked with your thyroid function, and adrenal fatigue and thyroid deficiency go hand in hand. Damaged or exhausted adrenals are unable to produce enough cortisol, which is necessary for thyroid hormone production, conversion of T4 to T3, and receptor function. Conversely, if your thyroid isn't functioning well, the slowdown this causes in your metabolism slows your adrenal function as well. If your thyroid and adrenal glands aren't healthy, when your levels of estrogen and progesterone decrease it's impossible for your body to function well and you will most likely feel miserable. Many doctors who treat thyroid disorders have theorized that almost 80 percent of women with low thyroid function also suffer from adrenal fatigue. Unfortunately, the shift to a more drug-driven approach to disease has obscured this knowledge. Doctors rarely look at the relationship between adrenal and thyroid function. But if you have symptoms of low thyroid, it's always good to evaluate your adrenal function as well. If your adrenals aren't producing enough cortisol, you should speak to your doctor about starting on low-dose cortisol supplementation at the same time as you add thyroid hormones.

Things to Remember

- Hypothyroidism is often hard to detect. Thyroid lab tests are notoriously inaccurate and "normal" ranges have proven to be only general indicators of dysfunction. If your symptoms are strongly suggestive of low thyroid function, sometimes the only course open to you and your doctor is for you to start on a trial course of thyroid hormone replacement and see if you respond.
- Finding the best treatment for hypothyroidism generally involves a trial-and-error process to determine what hormone therapy is optimal for each individual. The most common therapy, supplementing T4, isn't optimal for many women, as they may have difficulty converting T4 into T3, the more active form of thyroid hormone. If this is the case, you'll need to try a combination T4 and T3 therapy. Armour Thyroid is an excellent choice for initial thyroid therapy.
- Your thyroid and adrenal functions are closely intertwined, and you shouldn't start treatment for deficiency in one without having your levels of both thyroid hormones and cortisol evaluated. If levels of both are low, replacement of both hormones should be done concurrently.

CHAPTER 6

Out of Steam: *Adrenal Imbalance*

Joan's Story

Until she was forty-three-years old, Joan was active and energetic. A single parent with a twelve-year-old daughter and a ten-year-old son, she started every morning with a 5 a.m. run. This kept her in shape and gave her the energy she needed to be a good parent and keep on top of her demanding career as a regional sales manager for a large telecommunications company, a job that required frequent travel and long hours, including working on weekends.

But a few months after her forty-third birthday, things began to change. Although neither her diet nor her exercise routine had changed,

Joan was getting heavier, especially around her waist. She'd always heard that metabolic rates slow down with age, so she assumed this was what was happening to her and decided to fight it by adding a mile to her daily run and cutting back her evening wine to one glass. Unfortunately, this didn't help, and soon she began feeling tired and listless, just wanting to lie down at three in the afternoon and call it a day. She started drinking more coffee, and for the first time in her life she began craving high-carb, sugary foods, which did give her more energy but also created an addictive cycle. She ended up gaining more weight, which added self-loathing to the depression she was starting to feel and the stress she already suffered.

Things deteriorated slowly over the next few years as Joan steadily lost her stamina. She desperately wanted to feel like her old self again and tried everything from vitamin supplements to yoga, but nothing helped. Then, when she was forty-seven, she suffered a debilitating case of pneumonia over the Christmas holidays. She'd never been so sick in her life, and it took her weeks to get back on her feet. The same thing happened the next two years as well, always over the Christmas holidays, and each year it took her longer to recover. After her third and most severe bout of pneumonia, Joan was out of commission for six weeks. Then she returned to work too soon, which caused an additional five-week relapse.

Joan was lucky to find a doctor who suspected that adrenal fatigue was the cause of her health problems. She recommended a thorough physical, including a saliva test that measured her cortisol levels at 8 a.m., 12 noon, 4 p.m., and 10 p.m. The results showed that Joan's cortisol profile was a lower-than-normal morning peak, then an almost immediate drop in levels with virtually no cortisol production in the afternoon and evening. These findings were consistent with Joan's report of a noticeable drop in energy in the afternoon and severe fatigue in the evening.

Joan's doctor started her on 20 mg of cortisol per day for three months to start the process of rebuilding her adrenals. Her doctor also suggested specific lifestyle changes for Joan, including an eating plan that included protein and complex carbohydrates and limited her intake of caffeine, white flour, alcohol, and sugar.

At the end of the three months of treatment, Joan felt great. She followed her doctor's recommendation and suspended her cortisol use for one week to see whether she had built up enough adrenal function to stop the cortisol supplementation. She became very fatigued again and her test results showed she still had significantly low cortisol levels. Joan and her doctor decided to continue her low-dose cortisol supplementation for another six months, and Joan also continued the lifestyle changes. She had found that after several weeks of cortisol replacement and her new diet, she was no longer craving caffeine, alcohol, and simple carbohydrates. She was able to cut back to one cup of coffee in the morning and no alcohol at all in the evenings. Eventually, her energy returned to levels she hadn't experienced since she was in her early thirties.

THE IMPORTANCE OF THE ADRENALS

Like so many other women, Joan was able to function well until her estrogen and progesterone levels dropped significantly during her forties. Then she couldn't keep up the juggling act. If your lifestyle is demanding, sometimes getting hit with an illness (or injury or pregnancy) causes your body to screech to a halt and simply refuse to keep going. When your adrenals reach this stage of exhaustion, fixing them isn't as simple as just changing your diet or exercise routine, although these are important ingredients in an overall wellness plan. Cortisol, the critical adrenal hormone responsible for managing your body's stress, should be measured as soon as possible to determine your levels.

Adrenal fatigue is a huge problem today, and it's almost always caused or compounded by cumulative stressful emotional or physical events, although it can sometimes be tracked to one major event, such as an accident. The great news, however, is that this condition can be treated and reversed, no matter what stage you're at when it's diagnosed.

Your adrenal glands are vital to your health. They're responsible for the regulation of your body's balance of water and minerals; metabolism (utilization and distribution of carbohydrates, protein, and fat); allergic and immune reactions, including autoimmune diseases; and production of hormones (progesterone, testosterone, estrogens, and more). They also produce adrenaline and cortisol, incredibly powerful hormones that manage emotional and physical stress and produce a burst of energy to fuel the fight-or-flight response in the face of stress or danger. In earlier times, this was critical for surviving marauding animals, unfriendly tribes, or other threats to your survival. If you were in danger, your adrenal glands kicked in, you dealt with the situation, and then—if you survived—you went back to grinding maize or tending your baby, with plenty of time to recover before the next emergency.

Today, our lives are filled with different kinds of threats. From the moment our alarm clock wakes us up, we're bombarded with continual stressors all day long: traffic jams, household chores, kids' schedules, and unending bills. This may sound preferable to fighting off enemies or wild animals intent on eating us, but the truth is, stress is stress no matter what the cause, and if you don't manage it, it takes a toll on your health.

The human body was biologically designed for the short-term physical stress of immediate danger, not long-term psychological stress. We go through a preprogrammed response to stress of any kind: Heart rate, blood pressure, body temperature, and breathing rate all increase. Levels of fat and sugar in the bloodstream also rise, which increases muscle strength and energy and sharpens your thinking to deal with the crisis. On the other hand, inessential activities are shut down: Blood vessels constrict in noncritical areas such as the feet, scalp, intestines, and hands, and digestion slows. Unfortunately, the body responds in basically the same way to a complaining teenager as it does to marauding hordes.

When stressors continually bombard the adrenals, they produce ongoing high levels of cortisol. If your bodily functions return to normal quickly after the stressful situation is resolved, all is well. However, when you can't escape the stressor or manage it through diet and exercise, the continually elevated cortisol levels that result can cause unpleasant symptoms: ulcers, high blood pressure, depression, anxiety, heart disease, fatigue, weight gain, food or alcohol cravings, memory problems, and frequent illnesses. If you don't watch out, an extended period of this abnormal activity can cause your adrenals to become fatigued. Then they'll produce lower and lower levels of cortisol and you'll be increasingly less able to deal with stress of any kind. It's interesting to note that most people with clinical depression also have a cortisol imbalance, suggesting that chronic stress and depression do indeed go hand in hand. Once optimal adrenal function is restored, most of the conditions listed above will resolve.

When the ovaries' production of hormones slows down, and finally stops at menopause, the adrenals take over and become your major source of sex hormones.

When you consider the many critical functions of estrogen, progesterone, and testosterone, you can see how important this backup supply is. But if your adrenals are worn out, they certainly won't be able to make adequate levels of sex hormones, let alone handle stress effectively.

Your adrenal health depends on many factors beyond the number of stressful incidents you experience, including what kind of food you eat; what vitamins and minerals you take; how much you exercise, sleep, and rest; your overall hormone balance, including thyroid and ovarian function; your attitudes; your support network of friends and family; and your faith. All of these add up to determine how resistant or susceptible you are to stress and adrenal overload.

HOW CORTISOL INTERACTS WITH OTHER HORMONES

Adrenal, thyroid, and ovarian hormones must work together, and their interaction is as important as their individual functions. Elevated levels of cortisol interrupt this balance and cause the body to become resistant to other hormones, which means your tissues won't respond normally to estrogen and progesterone signals even if levels of those hormones are normal. High cortisol also blocks estrogen and progesterone activity and causes their levels to drop, resulting in infrequent ovulation. This puts further strain on the adrenals, since they now have to produce the progesterone that should have been produced as a result of ovulation.

Cortisol is also critical for your body to effectively use thyroid hormones: Low thyroid and low adrenal function go hand in hand. If you have low cortisol and you start on thyroid therapy, the thyroid hormones can increase your metabolism and thus speed the rate at which cortisol is cleared from your body. If your adrenal glands aren't functioning well, you won't be able to replace cortisol fast enough, so you'll end up with a cortisol deficiency, making you feel worse (Honeyman-Lowe and Lowe 2003).

How Healthy Is Your Liver?

Your thyroid ensures that your liver works well enough to use and excrete cortisol effectively. If your thyroid and, subsequently, your liver, is malfunctioning, cortisol levels will build up in your body even if overall production is low. But one serious illness or stressful event can deplete this supply of excess cortisol. When this occurs, your fatigued adrenals won't be able to produce cortisol fast enough to meet your body's ongoing needs, and this can precipitate a health crisis.

Your body may be sending you signals that your liver isn't functioning at its best, but you may not recognize them for what they are. Any of the following symptoms are indicators that low thyroid function may be affecting your liver's performance:

- Heightened sensitivity to medications
- Digestive problems, such as indigestion or reflux
- Pain in or near your liver if you press on it
- Coated tongue
- Dark circles under your eyes
- Yellowish skin or whites of the eyes
- Golden brown rings around your irises

Here's an easy way to check your liver function: Begin by leaning forward and breathing out. Next, take the four fingers of your right hand and push them up under the bottom of the right side of your rib cage. If you feel pain when you do this, your liver and/or gallbladder may not be functioning well. You should be able to fit your fingers in at least to the second knuckle. If you can't, your liver may be swollen, in which case you should talk to your doctor about getting a liver function test. Fixing this can be as easy as changing your diet, or it may signal a thyroid deficiency or some other condition.

What I Learned

After several false starts, I finally arrived at the right dose and type of thyroid therapy (two grains of Armour Thyroid daily) and felt great within two days. When I felt great for two weeks, I thought all my problems were over. About the time I started thinking I was finally completely well, my symptoms started coming back. I got very tired in the afternoons again, my thinking wasn't as clear as it had been, and my vision started to blur. Knowing now that it was possible to be completely well, I continued my research and came across the adrenal connection, which convinced me that my adrenals were exhausted and not making adequate cortisol.

I realized that when I started to replace thyroid hormones, my metabolism increased, triggering my liver to function normally for the first time in years. Before long, all the backed up stores of cortisol that had been circulating in my body due to inadequate liver clearance were finally used up, and I was left with an immediate deficiency of cortisol, which made me feel worse. I had my cortisol levels and profile measured, and the results showed that I had extremely low cortisol levels throughout the day. I started on 5 mg of bioidentical cortisol (Cortef, or hydrocortisone) four times a day (20 mg per day) and felt completely well again.

As my story illustrates, if you have low thyroid hormone levels, low adrenal function can be a huge compounding issue. Treating your thyroid alone will often not resolve your symptoms, or it may resolve them only for a very short period of time. You might conclude that the thyroid therapy isn't working and stop the treatment, but then you'll end up back where you started—feeling tired and unwell.

I'm convinced that this thyroid-adrenal relationship was at the root of all my problems and started the downward spiral that ended with a diagnosis of MS. These two functions are so intertwined that they can precipitate a severe decline in all metabolic functions, and I believe this can mimic degenerative disease. This is not to say that there aren't other causes of these diseases. However, because of my experiences, I urge anyone with prolonged ill health, including chronic fatigue and fibromyalgia, as well as other, less debilitating conditions, to evaluate these two functions.

HOW MUCH CORTISOL DO YOU NEED?

Cortisol levels rise and fall over a twenty-four-hour period, as seen in the graph below. Levels are highest in the first hour after you wake up in the morning (for most of us between 6 a.m. and 8 a.m.) then drop sharply until 11 a.m. Levels decline gradually throughout the rest of the day and hit bottom between midnight and 2 a.m. This pattern can be affected when your adrenals are either too active or not active enough.

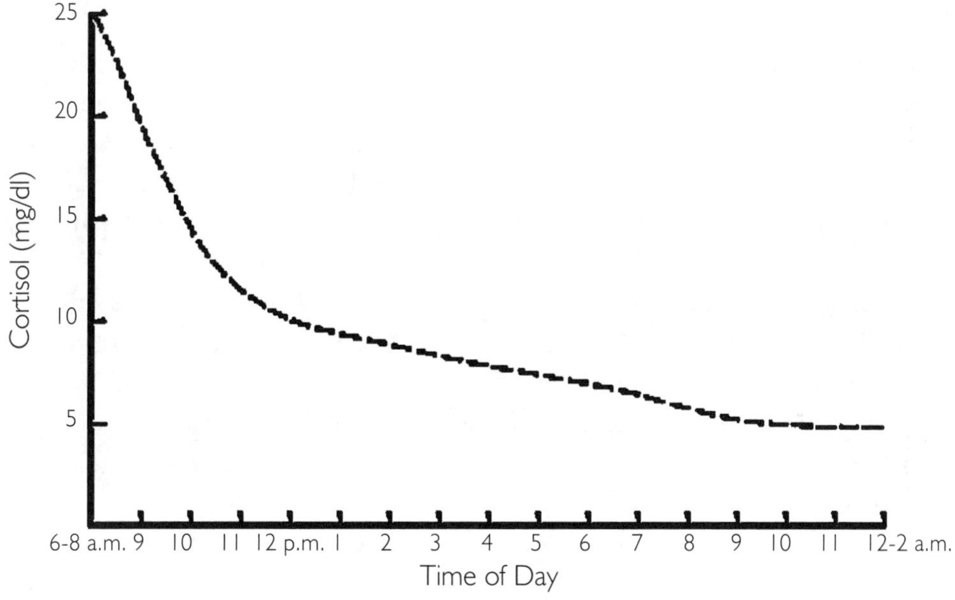

Daily Cortisol Production

It's possible for cortisol production to become too high, too low, or disrupted. When it's disrupted, you may miss the early morning peak and have a hard time getting started. That's when you find yourself increasing your intake of coffee or tea. Or if you have a high early morning level that drops precipitously later in the day, you'll feel extreme fatigue in the afternoon and have problems sleeping at night.

Disruption may also result in a reversed pattern—low cortisol levels in the morning, rising throughout the day and peaking in the afternoon or evening. This can cause you to have a surge of energy in the late afternoon or early evening and then be unable to sleep at night. Studies have shown that nighttime cortisol levels for a fifty-year-old are on average ten to twelve times higher than for a thirty-year-old, resulting in a lack of deep, restful sleep. In a vicious cycle, the resultant stress pushes levels of cortisol even higher (Laughlin and Barret-Connor 2000). These disrupted patterns create higher levels of cortisol, glucose, cholesterol, and insulin, along with elevated blood pressure, heart disease, diabetes, and weight gain.

When Your Cortisol Is Too High

The accelerated pace of our world these days can create chronic tension, anxiety, and exhaustion, which in turn causes excessive cortisol production. Stress (and yet more cortisol) can also be caused by physical catalysts, such as overexercising, overworking, a low-grade infection, or even continual irritation to your body from things such as mercury leaking from silver fillings in your teeth, high heavy metal levels in your body, or food allergies.

Besides stress, declining estrogen levels are one of the major catalysts of higher cortisol. Early signs that your cortisol may be elevated are food cravings, anxiety, and heart palpitations. At this stage, doctors generally prescribe antidepressants, which may help relieve the symptoms but do nothing for the cause. If this happens to you, I encourage you to persevere and get your adrenal function tested. Find out what's going on and cure the problem, don't just treat the symptoms.

You don't want to let this situation progress. Excess cortisol can impair your immune system and increase your blood pressure, cholesterol levels, triglyceride levels, osteoporosis risk, blood sugar levels, and insulin resistance. Insulin resistance leads to elevated glucose and insulin levels, and constant overexposure to these two powerful substances desensitizes your body to their effects, triggering it to make even more glucose (blood sugar). This vicious cycle can lead to weight gain, diabetes, and heart disease. Unexplained weight gain coupled with skin tags (small flaps of skin generally on the back of the neck or under the arms) is a good indicator of insulin resistance, indicating that testing should be pursued.

Unchecked insulin resistance can also lead to *syndrome X*, also known as metabolic syndrome. This condition is characterized by a cluster of metabolic problems that appear together, including insulin resistance, obesity primarily in the middle of the body, high cholesterol (and usually high triglycerides), and high blood pressure.

It's easy to see why women are at risk for this condition when you understand that it's triggered by high cortisol, which can in turn be triggered by dropping estrogen levels.

The first step in reducing cortisol levels is to lower insulin resistance through changes in your diet and exercise program. Cut back on white flour and sugar products, eat smaller, more frequent meals, cut out excessive salt, reduce alcohol use, and exercise regularly.

The Benefits of Exercise

Exercise is one of the best things you can do for your physical and mental well-being. Beyond helping to balance your adrenals, it can benefit you in many other ways, just a few of which are listed in the table below (Fletcher et al. 1996). As you'll see in this partial list, many of the benefits address common signs and symptoms of hormonal imbalance.

Exercise Helps You . . .	
Look your best.	Helps control weight and maintain optimal body weight and composition. Decreases body fat. Boosts testosterone production, which promotes muscle growth.
Feel your best.	Promotes psychological well-being. Reduces feelings of depression and anxiety. Increases self-esteem and self-confidence. Provides a break from your daily routine and worries.
Think your best.	Increases blood flow, which is critical to brain function. Relaxes and revitalizes. Reduces mental and muscular tension and, at the same time, increases concentration and energy level.

Be your healthiest.	Normalizes insulin levels and decreases risk of diabetes. Reduces the risk of colon cancer. Shuts down the stress response, which results in lower cortisol production; lowers blood pressure, blood sugar, and heart rate; and increases digestion, blood flow to skin, and production of growth hormone. Reduces the risk of developing high blood pressure and helps reduce blood pressure in people who already have high blood pressure. Raises levels of "good" cholesterol and lowers levels of "bad" cholesterol.

If you need any further encouragement to begin exercising, consider the following additional benefits of regular exercise: Inactive people are twice as likely to develop high blood pressure as active people, and fit women have diabetes much less often than unfit women. Exercise helps build and maintain healthy bones, muscles, and joints, and because it increases strength and balance, it reduces risks of falls and fractures. Regular exercise delays bone loss and promotes bone formation and thus decreases risk of osteoporosis. It also helps keep joints flexible and helps build muscle to support the joint, which can bring relief from arthritis symptoms.

EXERCISE: Assessing Symptoms of Excess Cortisol

The symptoms listed below are associated with excessive levels of cortisol. Check any that apply to you:

- ☐ Abdominal weight gain
- ☐ Anxiety
- ☐ Bloating and fluid retention
- ☐ Brain fog and memory problems
- ☐ Diabetes
- ☐ Food cravings
- ☐ High blood pressure
- ☐ Hypoglycemia
- ☐ Increased appetite
- ☐ Insomnia and sleep problems
- ☐ Irritability
- ☐ Loss of scalp hair
- ☐ Loss of sex drive
- ☐ Memory problems
- ☐ Muscle weakness and wasting
- ☐ Skin problems (thin skin, easy bruising, poor wound healing)
- ☐ Stomach problems (ulcers, irritable bowel syndrome, gastroesophageal reflux)
- ☐ Weight gain (fat buildup)

In your journal, write down all of the symptoms you checked, using the format in the example below. Note any details, such as when you first got the symptom, how long you've had it, and whether it's getting worse or better. Can you remember any trigger or event that may have precipitated the symptom, such as pregnancy or an accident or injury?

Symptom	When It Began and Precipitating Events	Getting Worse or Better?
I'm developing a layer of fat around my middle section and have uncontrollable food cravings.	*It started a couple of months ago, in May 2006. My husband and I had recently split up, and I've also been having a very stressful time at work.*	*Worse*

When Your Cortisol Is Too Low: Adrenal Fatigue

After your adrenals have produced chronic excessive cortisol to get you through the busy years of your thirties and forties, they may start to wear out, leaving you with adrenal fatigue. Adrenal fatigue can be caused by a sudden single event, such as a serious accident, the death of a loved one, or a divorce, but it's usually the result of years of cumulative physical and/or emotional stress. Lifestyle also plays an important part in how well you withstand stress; the amount and quality of sleep and rest you get, the dietary choices you make, and whether you have substance-abuse issues are all major considerations.

In the first phase of adrenal fatigue, your body produces enough cortisol for everyday activities, but not enough reserves to handle stressful situations. You may notice that even low-level stress or conflict leaves you feeling ill or shaken. A simple cold can seem to last forever. You weaken and become ultrasensitive, even to changes in temperature. A common catalyst for adrenal fatigue is chronic or severe infections, such as pneumonia, bronchitis, or chronic bouts of asthma, sinusitis, or respiratory infections. (Recurrent respiratory infections are almost always a sign of low adrenal function.) This is a vicious cycle, because every stressful situation depletes a little more of your adrenal reserves, causing even lower adrenal function and worsening symptoms.

For most women, the final blow to the adrenals is when estrogen and progesterone levels drop during perimenopause. We can handle almost anything when our ovarian hormone levels are high. In our thirties we manage kids, careers, relationships, marriages, or divorces with aplomb. But when we hit perimenopause and estrogen and progesterone levels decline, we become much more susceptible to stress, and even little things become overwhelming. Finally, our adrenals are further taxed as they take over production of ovarian hormones when the ovaries start to sputter. This is one of the reasons why bioidentical HRT can make so much sense for many of us.

The most extreme form of adrenal deficiency is Addison's disease. This condition, which afflicted John F. Kennedy, is often caused by autoimmune destruction of the adrenal gland, but it may have other causes, such as tuberculosis. Many other conditions are thought to be caused by adrenal fatigue as well, including fibromyalgia, hypoglycemia, alcoholism, depression, rheumatoid arthritis, ischemic heart disease, poor sleep, excessive sugar or caffeine consumption, respiratory infections, and chronic fatigue, pain, or asthma. If you have any of these conditions, find a doctor who specializes in adrenal health for a complete evaluation.

EXERCISE: Assessing Causes of Adrenal Fatigue

Here's a list of some of the more common events that can cause stress and contribute to adrenal fatigue. Check any that you've experienced:

- ☐ A major move
- ☐ Abusive spouse
- ☐ Assault
- ☐ Car accident
- ☐ Childbirth
- ☐ Chronic juggling of multiple roles at home and work
- ☐ Death of a spouse or loved one
- ☐ Divorce
- ☐ Extramarital affair (you or your spouse)
- ☐ Job change or loss
- ☐ Major change in diet
- ☐ Major change in living conditions
- ☐ Major change in sleeping habits
- ☐ Major change in social activities or friends
- ☐ Major illness
- ☐ Marriage
- ☐ Natural disaster
- ☐ Ongoing high pressure at work
- ☐ Pregnancy
- ☐ Retirement
- ☐ Separation
- ☐ Serious illness or accident (you or a close family member)
- ☐ Serious or chronic financial problems
- ☐ Sexual difficulties
- ☐ Significant loneliness
- ☐ Significant promotion
- ☐ Son or daughter leaving home
- ☐ Unhappy marriage or relationship
- ☐ Other serious emotional trauma: ____________________

In your journal, use the format in the example below to record any thoughts about the events you checked that can clarify their impact on your health. Also think about whether you had any change in your health around the time of these events. Did you notice any additional symptoms or were you diagnosed with any diseases or health conditions around that time?

Event	When It Occurred	Health Changes Around the Time of the Event
Car accident	*June 2002*	*Started having trouble sleeping and became depressed and tired much of the time.*

EXERCISE: Assessing Symptoms of Adrenal Fatigue

The symptoms listed below are associated with adrenal fatigue. Check any that apply to you:

- ☐ Abdominal pain
- ☐ Alcoholism
- ☐ Allergies
- ☐ Anxiety or panic attacks
- ☐ Asthma
- ☐ Back and groin pain
- ☐ Bowel problems
- ☐ Chronic or severe infections or illnesses
- ☐ Cognitive confusion
- ☐ Cold hands and feet
- ☐ Cold sweats
- ☐ Craving salt or sweets
- ☐ Dark circles under your eyes
- ☐ Depression
- ☐ Diarrhea
- ☐ Difficulty in exercising
- ☐ Dry, thin skin
- ☐ Eczema or psoriasis
- ☐ Environmental sensitivities
- ☐ Excessive fatigue
- ☐ Eyes sensitive to light
- ☐ Fainting
- ☐ Feeling ill after chronic stress or a severe stressful event
- ☐ Feeling of shaking or shivering inside
- ☐ Headaches
- ☐ Heart palpitations
- ☐ Hissing noises in your ears
- ☐ Hyperactivity
- ☐ Hypoglycemia
- ☐ Increased incidence of autoimmune disease
- ☐ Insomnia and sleep problems
- ☐ Intolerance of cold or heat
- ☐ Irritable bowel syndrome

- ☐ Joint pain
- ☐ Looking older than your age
- ☐ Loss of body hair
- ☐ Low blood pressure, particularly when rising from lying down to standing up
- ☐ Low sex drive
- ☐ Memory problems
- ☐ Muscle and joint pain
- ☐ Muscle weakness
- ☐ Pain at the bottom of the back of the rib cage
- ☐ Pale face
- ☐ PMS
- ☐ Sluggishness in the morning
- ☐ Stiff neck
- ☐ Sunken cheeks or eyes
- ☐ Symptoms of low thyroid made worse by hormone supplementation
- ☐ Upset stomach
- ☐ Waking at night with other symptoms
- ☐ Weak, slow, or soft pulse
- ☐ Weight loss

In your journal, write down all of the symptoms you checked, using the format in the example below. Also note anything that would help your doctor understand your condition more clearly, such as when you first got the symptom and whether it generally gets better or worse at certain points during the day or during your menstrual cycle.

Symptom	**When It Began**	**When It Improves or Worsens**	**Other Comments**
Started craving sweets	*When my menstrual periods became irregular about 2 years ago at 43.*	*Gets worse in the second half of my cycle.*	*Some cycles I don't get it so bad. Maybe I'm still ovulating in these cycles?*
Brain fog	*At 35*	*Gets worse in the second half of my cycle.*	*Can't seem to find words or finish sentences.*

TESTING YOUR ADRENAL FUNCTION

The symptoms in the checklist above are all indicative of low adrenal function. Some of them may also have other causes (particularly low estrogen or thyroid). If you have several of these symptoms or one particularly bothersome one such as irritable bowel syndrome, you should have your adrenal function tested.

Self-Tests for Adrenal Function

If you're concerned about your adrenal function, there are several simple tests you can do at home to determine whether you have a problem. None of these will accurately gauge your cortisol levels though, so if you find signs of adrenal dysfunction, make arrangements with your doctor to get lab tests. The precise levels measured by lab tests are important in deciding how to proceed with treatment.

PUPIL-CONTRACTION TEST

In the early 1900s, it was discovered that the pupil is a very accurate indicator of low adrenal function. Adrenal function affects the pupil's ability to contract and stay contracted when the retina is exposed to light. If your adrenals are fatigued, your pupil won't be able to remain contracted, so it will dilate unnaturally. To do this test you'll need a flashlight, a mirror, and a watch. Here's what you do:

1. Go into a darkened room with a mirror on the wall.
2. Look into the mirror and then shine the flashlight across your eye from the side. Hold the flashlight with the light pointing toward your temple.
3. Watch your pupil in the mirror as the light shines across it. The pupil should contract and stay contracted as the light hits it. If, after a short period of time (two minutes or less) while shining the light, it starts to dilate, then contracts, then dilates, and doesn't stay contracted, you most likely have some level of adrenal fatigue. (Very mild fatigue may not show up.) Time these periods of dilation and record your results below.

Date	Seconds Dilated		Date	Seconds Dilated

Repeat this test every month for several months to see if any of the therapies you're implementing (diet, exercise, or HRT) are helping your adrenal function to recover.

BLOOD PRESSURE TEST

Adrenal fatigue is one of the primary causes of low blood pressure. If your blood pressure drops when you rise from lying down to standing up, you may have low adrenal function. Like the other at-home tests, this one is simple enough to do, but you will need a blood pressure monitor to do the test. Here's what you do:

1. Lie down and relax for five to ten minutes.
2. Take your blood pressure while you're still lying down and write it down in your journal.
3. Stand up and take your blood pressure again. Note it in your journal.
4. When you stand, your blood pressure should go up about 10 mm Hg.

If your blood pressure drops when you stand, you may have adrenal fatigue, but you'll need to pursue other tests to confirm this.

WHITE LINE TEST

Adrenal fatigue was recognized as far back as 1917 by Emile Sergent, a French doctor. He developed a simple test that you can do at home using a ballpoint pen. Using the end opposite the pen point, make a mark about six inches long across your abdomen without pressing hard or scratching the skin. If your adrenals are functioning normally, the mark will turn from white to red fairly rapidly. If your adrenals are fatigued, after about a minute you'll begin to notice a pale line, which will become white, more distinct, and, eventually, wider than the original line. It will be most visible in about one minute, then fade after about three minutes. A drawback to this test is that only about 40 percent of people with low adrenal function test positive, but if you do test positive, it's almost certain that you have low adrenal function (Harrower 1922).

Lab Tests for Adrenal Function

If you have several of the symptoms of adrenal fatigue listed above, particularly severe fatigue, it's important to have your cortisol levels tested. You and your doctor can't come up with an effective treatment plan until you know what your levels are and assess your adrenal function. If your cortisol levels are abnormal, you can gather additional information about how your adrenals are functioning by testing levels of a couple of other hormones: adrenocorticotropic hormone (ACTH) and aldosterone (more on these hormones below).

CORTISOL LEVELS

Cortisol levels can be assessed by blood tests, urine tests, or saliva tests, any of which can be ordered by your doctor. The saliva and urine tests are kits that your doctor will either give to you or have shipped to you. They come with directions for how to collect the samples, complete with an airbill to mail the samples back to the lab. The most widely accepted test for cortisol is still the blood test. This is a very accurate test, but it requires you to go to the lab at least twice in one day to have blood drawn. The saliva test is very convenient as samples may be collected anywhere, even at work, whereas the twenty-four-hour urine test would need to be done on a day when you can stay close to the collection container. Although the saliva test is promising, it hasn't been used for a very long period of time yet, so many doctors aren't comfortable using it. Your doctor will most likely have a preference for one type of testing methodology, and all three have both pros and cons.

Blood test: To get a completely accurate picture of your twenty-four-hour profile, you'd have to go to the lab at 8 a.m., 12 noon, 4 p.m., and 10 p.m., which isn't practical. Most doctors will only test levels at 8 a.m. and 4 p.m. This test can be done on any day of your cycle.

Twenty-four-hour urine test: For this test, you collect all of your urine for a twenty-four-hour period. While this will show how much cortisol you produce, it doesn't detect patterns of production or a disrupted rhythm, which can also create health problems.

Saliva test: This measures your daily cyclic profile of cortisol production to determine if you have an abnormal pattern. Most doctors advocate a four-point saliva test, measuring levels at four points during the day: 8 a.m., 12 noon, 4 p.m., and 10 p.m. It will show if deficiency exists at any of these times, showing you have a disrupted production cycle that may lead to symptoms and health problems.

ACTH AND ALDOSTERONE TESTS

ACTH, a hormone produced by the pituitary, stimulates your adrenals to produce cortisol, so levels of this hormone are obviously critical to adrenal function. If your cortisol levels are low, it may be worthwhile to test ACTH to determine if the problem lies in the pituitary or in the adrenals. Because aldosterone is produced by the adrenals, levels of this hormone, as well as cortisol, can be used to gauge overall adrenal function.

ACTH blood test: This determines levels of ACTH, the hormone that stimulates the adrenals, to see whether the problem is with the pituitary or the adrenal glands. This test must be ordered by your doctor and may be done at anytime during your menstrual cycle.

ACTH challenge test: This test assesses adrenal reserves and is an indicator of adrenal fatigue. First, baseline cortisol levels are tested, then ACTH is injected. Cortisol is measured again after an hour to see how the adrenals responded. Your cortisol level should double.

Aldosterone levels: This is a simple blood test to assess levels of aldosterone, another hormone secreted by the adrenals, which is responsible for water and salt balance in the body. When your adrenals don't make enough aldosterone, fluid is pulled out of the tissues and skin, and this can cause your face and eyes to appear sunken. The drug Florinef (fludrocortisone) is used to correct inadequate levels of aldosterone.

TREATMENT OF ADRENAL FATIGUE

Doctors frequently overlook adrenal problems, whether overstimulation or fatigue. Although adrenal fatigue has been recognized for over a hundred years, doctors were more likely to look at your adrenal function in 1950 than they are today. This is part of the general trend in medicine, which is becoming increasingly specialized and moving away from the practice of looking at the whole body to find interconnected, underlying problems. In addition, medical schools in this country don't focus on adrenal fatigue, so even endocrinologists specializing in hormones rarely recognize the problem. This is why you must educate yourself about your adrenals, analyze your symptoms carefully, and be prepared to lay out the facts for your doctor. If your doctor isn't interested in analyzing your situation and helping you get to the bottom of it, you may have to look for a doctor with a background in diagnosing and treating adrenal problems. The first step is to find out what your cortisol levels are. If they're low, consider rebuilding them in one of the following ways.

Cortisol Replacement

Cortisol replacement is a valuable therapy for adrenal fatigue. Bioidentical cortisol replacement replenishes your natural reserves and returns them to normal levels. This relieves the stress on your adrenal glands, giving them time to relax and recover. Doctors always recommend starting with a low dose so as to not completely shut down your body's own production of cortisol. Normal daily production is around 35 to 40 mg per day, so most doctors will recommend starting with 20 mg or less.

Doctors recommend various dosing schedules depending on their past experience, your particular cortisol profile, and how you respond to the therapy. Some suggest four equal doses a day of 5 mg each at meals and bedtime. Other doctors prefer to mimic the body's normal production pattern and prescribe three doses a day, having you take the largest dose first thing in the morning, a smaller dose around noon, and the smallest and final dose at about 4 p.m.

Many doctors are unaware of, or uncomfortable with, prescribing bioidentical cortisol hormone replacement. It has been suggested that this is because they don't understand the difference between natural, bioidentical cortisol and cortisol that has been chemically altered, like prednisone and prednisolone, which have much more long-lasting effects on the body and dangerous side effects (Jefferies 1996).

Adrenal Extracts

Supplements made from bovine adrenal glands can also rebuild your adrenal glands. These natural adrenal extracts help to support and restore your adrenals by a somewhat different method than cortisol replacement: Rather than supplying cortisol, they strengthen your existing adrenal function, enhancing your adrenals' ability to produce cortisol on their own. They're a good alternative if your adrenals are still fairly functional. You can purchase adrenal extracts at most natural foods stores, or online from many sources.

Vitamins and Minerals

When you're experiencing adrenal fatigue, rebuilding your body with a well-balanced multivitamin and mineral supplement is very important. Supplements help prevent vitamin and mineral deficiencies when your diet doesn't provide all the necessary nutrients. But when your adrenal function is less than optimal, supplements are critical. The extra nutrients they supply enable your body to recover from vitamin and mineral deficiencies and any resulting compromised functions. Larger amounts of some nutrients are necessary for rebuilding adrenal function, especially all of the B vitamins, magnesium, zinc, and vitamin C.

Exercise

Although exercise is the last treatment method described here, it is by no means the least critical element in effectively managing stress and rebuilding your adrenals. Done regularly, even minimal exercise will help your body take stress in stride. Exercise prevents stressors from becoming cumulative and allows the body to escape the ill effects of chronic stress. And if you're still unconvinced, exercise increases blood flow and oxygen levels and normalizes levels of hormones, including thyroid, insulin, cortisol, and growth hormone. If you don't currently have an exercise routine, the best way to come up with one that you'll stick to is to find

Benefits of Walking

Walking is one of the best forms of exercise if you're just starting an exercise program. It helps reduce blood sugar by taking glucose out of your bloodstream and delivering it to your muscles. Other benefits include reducing the risk of chronic diseases, such as heart disease, high blood pressure, obesity, osteoporosis, non-insulin-dependent diabetes, and certain cancers. Results from the twenty-year Nurses' Health Study have shown significant decreases in occurrence of breast cancer and type 2 diabetes in women who engaged in brisk walking or other vigorous exercise for seven hours a week, and reductions in heart disease with as little as three hours a week. In this study, brisk walking was defined as 3 to 3.9 miles per hour, or fifteen to twenty minutes per mile (Manson et al. 1999).

Studies reveal that exercise has positive effects on emotional disorders, regardless of gender and age. The benefits are significant, especially for those with anxiety or depression. The greatest improvements are achieved through rhythmic aerobic exercises that use large muscle groups, such as walking. To achieve the full effects, you should exercise at least fifteen to thirty minutes at a time at least three times a week, and for at least ten weeks (Guszkowska 2004).

Another benefit of walking is that it stimulates your lymphatic system, which doesn't have a pump as your circulatory system does. Swinging your arms while walking pumps lymphatic fluid through your system. This fluid fills the spaces around all of your cells. After a cell digests its food, the waste is discharged into the lymph fluid. A system of vessels carries this waste to one of your large veins to be carried in your blood to your liver and other organs, which filter and clean it.

something you enjoy doing that fits with your lifestyle. Too many of us make rash decisions to join an expensive gym, or we sign up for a demanding class that we end up hating and subsequently not doing. Start simple. Walking with a friend is a great way to combine the best of both worlds; you'll enjoy the entertainment of chatting with a friend while also getting exercise.

RESTORING ADRENAL BALANCE

Whether you're producing too much or too little cortisol, adrenal imbalance can lead to serious health problems. Because doctors seldom suspect adrenal fatigue, they generally don't know to test cortisol levels and treat imbalances. Until this condition becomes better known in the medical community, each of us must be on the lookout for the signs and symptoms of adrenal imbalance and bring any evidence of this to the attention of our doctors.

If you're one of the millions who suffer from adrenal fatigue or adrenal overstimulation, regaining your health is within your grasp. The first step is to analyze your symptoms to see if they appear to be related to cortisol deficiency or excess. The next step is to find a doctor who understands adrenal evaluation and treatment and who will work with you to test and treat any problems detected. And the final step is to make easy but profound changes to your diet and lifestyle that will support any additional therapies, such as cortisol replacement. As indicated by Joan's story, at the start of this chapter, and as you learned in chapter 1, changing your diet to reduce your intake of sugars and refined carbohydrates will be immensely helpful. Reducing consumption of caffeine and alcohol is also a good idea. And please try to carve out some time for regular, moderate exercise. Though the time commitment may seem daunting, most people find that after a short time on an exercise program they have more energy and mental clarity. These benefits will probably free up more time than you spend exercising!

Things to Remember

- You may be making too much or too little cortisol. Either condition is bad and can seriously affect your thyroid function and overall health.
- Not only is it important that your overall level of cortisol isn't too high or too low, it's also critical that your pattern of production is optimal. Your levels should be highest first thing in the morning and gradually decrease throughout the day.
- When your estrogen level drops, your cortisol level rises, leading to problems such as abdominal weight gain and lack of insulin and glucose regulation. You should implement changes in diet and exercise to stop excess cortisol production. Also consider HRT to bolster deficient estrogen levels.
- Low-dose bioidentical cortisol is a useful therapy to rebuild low adrenal function.

CHAPTER 7

Out of Hormones: *Menopause*

Betsy's Story

Betsy had been a young-looking forty-seven-year-old, she was medium height and slender, with great skin and thick, shiny, shoulder-length hair. She'd felt so well and had such an easy time through her forties that she'd begun to think her friends who had already been through perimenopause had exaggerated their experiences just to scare her, the way some women had when she was pregnant with her first child, describing their twenty-nine hours of labor that ended in emergency Caesarean sections.

But midway through her forty-seventh year, Betsy's problems began. First there were the bladder infections, which were painful, continual, and seemingly impossible to cure. Then came the need to go to the bathroom four or five times every night, which deprived her of needed sleep. But what wasn't keeping her up at night anymore was sex; she'd lost every last bit of interest in it and didn't even have the energy or desire to go through the motions. Her husband tried his best to be patient and understanding, but since Betsy herself didn't understand what was happening to her, this was difficult and frustrating for both of them. And it seemed that many other things that used to be easy were now difficult and frustrating, including relationships with people she loved. She found herself often irritated by her teenage children, her husband, and even her friends.

On top of everything else, Betsy's body was changing in ways that made her feel unattractive and even a little frightened. She seemed to be losing muscle mass, and her breasts, face, and arms were getting skinny; she'd gone from slender to bony and haggard looking. Her mother and grandmother had become thinner as they'd aged, and to ward off the same fate Betsy had always worked out, lifting weights and taking step aerobics classes, but now these didn't seem to make much difference. Her shiny hair was growing dull and dry, and it even started breaking off when she brushed it. Her hairdresser suggested a shorter style to cope with it, which made her even more depressed when she looked around at all the middle-aged women with short, thinning hair. But the hot flashes were the last straw—the sudden intolerable waves of sweating and heat that hit her unexpectedly, debilitating and embarrassing her. This is what finally motivated Betsy to make an appointment with her doctor.

Fortunately, her doctor recognized that her symptoms were due to low estrogen and recommended checking her levels of follicle stimulating hormone and estrogen. Her FSH was 70 mIU/ml (million international units per milliliter; anything over 30 is considered a menopausal level) and her estradiol was 13 pg/ml (anything under 40 coupled with a high FSH level is considered menopausal). These results showed that Betsy was almost out of estrogen. Her doctor recommended a 0.1 mg estrogen patch (the strongest bioidentical FDA-approved concentration available) with progesterone in intravaginal form during the last two weeks of her cycle. Once Betsy started using the patch, she felt immediate relief from her symptoms, and as her doctor pointed out, she also had the benefit of added protection from osteoporosis and heart disease. Another side benefit she soon noticed was shine and life coming back into her hair and skin.

WHAT TO EXPECT AT MENOPAUSE

Unlike Betsy, some women have a fairly easy path through menopause. They experience the normal, unavoidable changes associated with dwindling estrogen levels, such as wrinkled, dry skin, vaginal dryness, worsening vision, and loss of breast fullness. But in areas that really count for quality of life—energy, libido, mood, ability to sleep, and freedom from pain—they're mostly fine. If you're one of these lucky women, hormonal intervention may be required only to ease symptoms during the immediate transition to menopause, or you may not require any treatment at all.

The next group may seem even luckier. They have no signs of low estrogen whatsoever. Their breasts remain full, their skin looks great, their vaginas don't lose tone or lubrication, and their minds and memories are as crisp as they were in their youth. The benefit these women enjoy comes from the very high levels of estrogen they've inherited. The drawback they face comes during perimenopause, when they no longer make adequate levels of progesterone to balance their robust levels of estrogen. And even after menopause, they're in an unbalanced hormone state, with too much estrogen relative to progesterone. However, in the world of hormone problems this is an easy thing to fix. If you're one of these lucky women, make sure to get your estrogen levels checked and to balance your estrogen with supplemental progesterone to prevent the symptoms and conditions associated with unbalanced estrogen (mood swings, sleeplessness, and increased risk of breast, endometrial, and uterine cancer). It's also wise to get a pelvic ultrasound to make sure you haven't experienced any buildup of the endometrial lining (caused by the proliferative effect of high estrogen levels), which can pose a potential cancer risk.

The final group of menopausal women has significant symptoms or health conditions (such as osteoporosis) that affect their health and ability to function normally. These are the women who have many of the severe symptoms of low estrogen listed below. Unless their levels of estrogen and progesterone are corrected, they will suffer a profoundly compromised quality of life. HRT can confer increased capability, strength, and vitality and thus significantly ease the aging process, improving their quality of life and preventing disease.

Estrogen Levels Decline

We usually start to notice declining estrogen levels through overt physical changes: Our hair gets dry and coarse and starts to thin, our contact lenses start hurting and causing problems, our vision starts to dim, our skin gets dry, our breasts start to flatten and sag, and we start to notice wrinkles at the corners of the nose, eyes, and mouth. As drastic as these changes in appearance may seem, they're really only the tip of the iceberg in terms of what's happening throughout our bodies. Estrogen and progesterone receptors are involved in critical functions everywhere, though their effects may be most obvious in our skin, scalp, and breasts. And once this transition begins, it progresses fairly rapidly—in fact, most women lose 90 percent of their estrogen in just two years. Here are some of the most troublesome symptoms that many women encounter at menopause:

- Brain fog and memory problems
- Decreased sex drive
- Deflated, sagging breasts
- Dry eyes
- Dry, thin skin
- Dry vagina
- Gum and tooth problems
- Hair loss
- Hot flashes
- Insomnia and sleep problems
- Irritability and mood swings
- Osteoporosis
- Painful intercourse
- Stiffness and pain
- Urinary incontinence or urgency
- Vision problems
- Weight gain

Take the time now to go back to the exercise "Assessing Symptoms of Deficient Estrogen" in chapter 4. That exercise contains a more complete list of the symptoms of estrogen deficiency. The primary difference between the symptoms of deficient estrogen in perimenopause and those at menopause is that symptom severity is generally worse at menopause. Also closely review everything you noted in your journal for that exercise. You might even want to do that exercise again, particularly if it's been a while since you worked on chapter 4, or if your awareness of your symptoms has changed as you've read forward from that point. If you experience several symptoms of deficient estrogen, particularly the physical ones such as hot flashes or bladder and vaginal problems, you most likely have fairly low levels of estrogen. Schedule an appointment with your doctor as soon as possible to review your symptoms and arrange for a thorough physical and the tests of hormone levels described in chapter 4. If your estrogen levels are low, HRT may be beneficial.

When you seek your doctor's help with these symptoms, you'll most likely be given a follicle stimulating hormone test, but it only tells part of the story. As your ovaries make less and less estrogen, your brain responds by increasing levels of FSH. If your FSH level is over 30 mIU/ml, you'll be pronounced menopausal. However, it's also crucial to test your levels of estrogen, progesterone, testosterone, and thyroid and adrenal hormones. These will tell the rest of the story. If estrogen and progesterone are balanced, albeit at a much lower level as evidenced by the end of your menstrual cycles, and your adrenal and thyroid functions are still robust, then sometimes supplementing deficient vitamins and minerals, combined with lifestyle and diet changes, is all that's needed to restore your health. You should work with your doctor to test and understand your levels of these key hormones.

The Telltale Signs of Menopause

There are several physical characteristics of menopause that you can spot from a distance. Perhaps the most universal is dry, fading hair. As soon as estrogen levels fall, a woman's hair gets thin, wispy, and dry; very few women retain the shiny hair of their youth. Another common characteristic of menopausal women is a thicker body. This is the body's way of naturally coping with estrogen loss. As you may recall from chapter 1, estrone, the type of estrogen that dominates after menopause, is made in fat cells, and it can buffer the discomfort of going through this hormonal transition by providing a backup supply of estrogen. A bit of fat is natural, and if you choose to not replace estradiol, it will ease your transition. But don't allow this to make you complacent about more significant weight gain. If your adrenal glands, thyroid, lifestyle, or diet gets out of control, you may become seriously overweight or obese. The heavier you are, the more estrone you'll produce, increasing the likelihood of additional health problems, including high blood sugar, diabetes, early heart attacks or strokes, slower blood circulation, higher free radical production, and increased risk of breast or uterine cancers.

Other menopausal changes are just as profound but harder to spot. One of the most relationship affecting is loss of sexual desire. Sexual desire ebbs and flows throughout life, and for most of us, libido naturally declines as we age. If your sex life is less active but still satisfying, you have absolutely nothing to worry about and should, in fact, count yourself lucky. On the other hand, if you've completely lost interest in sex or can no longer function as you usually have, consider undergoing a thorough physical to determine the cause of the problem. Balancing hormones could be a potential solution for you. Dr. Philip Sarrel, professor emeritus of obstetrics and gynecology at Yale University School of Medicine, determined that to have normal sexual function, women should have a blood estrogen level of at least 50 pg/ml (Sarrel 2000); not many women have such levels after menopause.

THE ROLE OF HORMONES IN WEIGHT

Though weight gain is just one symptom of hormonal imbalance, it's a problem that plagues many women, particularly after menopause. Imbalances or deficiencies of any of the hormones discussed in this book may result in weight gain, and the alarming statistic that 66 percent of American women over forty are overweight (Flegal et al. 2002) makes it impossible to ignore the fact that hormonal imbalance can be related to weight gain.

Here's the typical scenario women face when their hormones start to shift: Estrogen drops sometime after age thirty-five, causing cortisol to go up. The increasing cortisol suppresses estrogen even more, and also interferes with thyroid function. The extra fat produced by this high cortisol and low thyroid causes more estrone to be produced, which in turn makes more fat. Progesterone can also play a role in weight gain, as it causes food cravings when your levels are too high compared to dropping estrogen levels. Because of testosterone's importance in maintaining muscle mass, declining testosterone levels are involved, too. Let's take a closer look at the role of each of these hormones in weight gain.

Estrogen

When estrogen drops, it affects your weight in several ways and causes several things to occur simultaneously. Your body increases its production of estrone, the postmenopause estrogen that's produced in fat cells. But estrone fuels a vicious cycle: The extra fat you develop actually produces its own estrone, leading to even more fat. Decreasing estrogen also results in higher cortisol levels, leading to insulin resistance and more storage of fat around your middle. And as your testosterone-to-estrogen ratio becomes higher as a result of decreased estrogen, this results in a male pattern of fat distribution. So your fat gravitates from your hips and thighs to your stomach, and you lose your hourglass shape.

Declining estrogen also causes muscle loss and decreased muscle tone, which is unfortunate because muscle is a key weapon in the fat-burning arsenal. The more muscle you have, the more fat you burn. You can't go by your scales alone at this time of life, since muscle weighs much more than fat. If you're losing muscle and gaining fat, your scale will tell you you're holding steady even if you're seeing a drastic change for the worse in your shape. Estrogen loss can have other negative impacts on your muscles because it increases loss of key minerals, such as potassium (Aloia et al. 1991), calcium, magnesium, and zinc. Potassium is needed for healthy muscle, and calcium, magnesium, and zinc are required for optimal metabolism and muscle functioning.

Sufficient estrogen is also critical to the restorative deep stage of sleep. When your estrogen levels drop, you'll have restless, fragmented sleep, which decreases your body's ability to stimulate muscle growth and repair. The resultant decrease in muscle mass leads to diminished ability to burn fat and, again, results in weight gain. Another result of insufficient sleep is reduced production of growth hormone, which also leads to loss of lean muscle and increased body fat. Finally, estrogen is required for optimal thyroid function, so when your estrogen levels drop, your thyroid function decreases and weight gain can result.

Progesterone

Progesterone causes an increase in hunger and food cravings. Many women find that their appetite increases and that they get overpowering food cravings in the last two weeks of their cycle, when progesterone is high. As estrogen levels drop with age, these symptoms may become even more pronounced. When you have too much progesterone relative to estrogen, either through supplementation or because of dropping estrogen levels, your body experiences a condition much like pregnancy (the only other time women have disproportionately high levels of progesterone). If you're pregnant, your body is oriented toward nurturing and protecting a baby, so you have more fat storage, slowed digestion, higher cortisol levels, and decreased sensitivity to glucose. This alteration in blood sugar regulation is why women have sugar cravings during pregnancy, and during the second half of the menstrual cycle, when progesterone is dominant.

Cortisol

Cortisol levels go up when estrogen drops. Since high cortisol levels also make your body less sensitive to estrogen and thyroid hormones, your remaining levels of these hormones can't be used effectively. These higher levels of cortisol create insulin resistance, which causes refined carbohydrates and sugars to be converted to fat instead of being burned as fuel. Eating these foods triggers a chain reaction, causing glucose, or blood sugar, to spike and then crash, making your body ravenous for all the wrong foods. This vicious cycle can cause compromised immune function, increased risk of heart disease and type 2 diabetes, and weight gain. This fat is almost always stored around the middle of your body.

If you've attempted to resolve your insulin resistance condition through diet and exercise and haven't been successful, you may want to consider the prescription drug Glucophage (metformin), which improves glucose tolerance and resolves insulin imbalance. It was traditionally used for diabetes patients, but it's now being used for people with serious insulin imbalances, such as women who are insulin-resistant because of various hormone imbalances combined with years of a diet high in simple carbohydrates. Sometimes it's the only thing that will reverse the insulin resistance and allow the body to right itself. It's particularly helpful for women who have polycystic ovary syndrome (PCOS), where insulin resistance is always involved.

Thyroid

Thyroid function diminishes when production of estrogen in the ovaries slows, causing a drop in all metabolic functions and resulting in weight gain. Your thyroid can also cause problems if you diet drastically, because your body believes you're starving and goes into the mode of storing everything. It does this by binding up T3 hormone with thyroid-binding hormone, which slows down your metabolism even more. This is why you get signs of hypothyroidism, such as dry skin, constipation, hair loss, and feeling cold and tired, shortly after starting a severely restricted diet. Thyroid hormones are also critical to your muscles, and when your levels are low, you're unable to build and maintain muscle. With low thyroid, you also won't get enough oxygen, which results in muscle pain, stiffness, and weakness, affecting your ability to exercise.

Testosterone

Testosterone levels also drop when ovarian function slows. Testosterone is critical to maintenance of muscles and muscle tone. When your testosterone level declines, your muscles will start to shrink and atrophy even if you continue to exercise. With diminished testosterone levels, you'll have a harder time building new muscle and keeping existing muscles strong. Your fat distribution will also change, with more fat developing particularly on your abdomen.

Too much testosterone can also be problematic. When your estrogen levels decrease, one result is lowered levels of SHBG (sex hormone binding globulin), which controls levels of androgens, including testosterone, available to your body. As a result, some women have more testosterone available in their body, causing it to take on more of an apple shape, with the weight collecting on the trunk and waist, and less of an estrogen-driven hourglass shape. This "apple" body type, with fat stored in the upper body, indicates a greater risk for heart disease and diabetes.

The Insulin Connection

You may be surprised to learn that insulin is a hormone. But with the ever-increasing numbers of women who are overweight and have type 2 diabetes at middle age, insulin is clearly an important hormone to watch as you near menopause. Produced by the pancreas, insulin is crucial for regulation of blood sugar levels. If you recall that all of the hormones in the endocrine system are interrelated, then you're well on your way to understanding that what you eat can affect your hormone levels, and that hormone imbalances might impact how your body responds to different foods.

Let's take a quick look at carbohydrates: There are two different types of carbohydrates. Simple carbohydrates are made up of single sugar molecules or two sugar molecules joined together. Complex carbohydrates are also made up of sugars, but the sugar molecules are strung together to form longer, more complex chains. Complex carbohydrates, such as grains, vegetables, peas, and beans, have a higher fiber content. When complex carbohydrates are consumed in the form of whole foods, they convert more slowly to glucose, which results in the release of less insulin, and at a slower pace.

However, many of these benefits are lost when foods are refined and processed, stripping them of their fiber-rich outer covering and, in the case of grains, removing the nutrient-rich germ. Once refined, complex carbohydrates convert to blood sugar, or glucose, much more quickly. Your muscle cells store this glucose (in the form of glycogen) until they get full. When this happens, these cells refuse to accept any more glucose, so your body stores it in fat cells to try to get it out of circulation. When your body releases more insulin to try to manage additional glucose, your blood sugar plunges, leading to blood sugar swings that cause cravings for sugar, simple carbs, and caffeine. It's simple: The more refined carbohydrates you eat, the more insulin you produce, and the more insulin you produce, the fatter you get. The bottom line is that eating too many refined carbohydrates leads to weight gain, particularly around your middle.

Try to avoid anything with sugar or white flour in it, such as candy, soft drinks, cookies, cake, pastries, doughnuts, and even fruit juices, as well as any breads, pasta, or cereals made with white flour. Instead focus on whole grains, such as brown rice, oatmeal, and breads and other products made from whole grains. The size of your meals and their timing are also important factors. Keep portions smaller and eat more often, never skip meals, and try to avoid eating a lot at night, because this causes more insulin production, leading to higher fat storage. Alcohol also stimulates insulin production and results in swings in blood sugar levels, so it's best to cut back as much as possible or avoid it altogether.

As you learned in chapter 6, adrenal dysfunction, which sometimes results from declining estrogen, can also create elevated insulin levels. So if your adrenals are fatigued, reducing your consumption of sugar and refined carbohydrates can ease the burden on your body.

Ellen's Story

When she was forty-five, a sudden onset of severe abdominal pain sent Ellen to the emergency room. After preliminary tests, an ultrasound revealed that she had several fibroids. Her gynecologist recommended removal of the fibroids, as well as her uterus. Ellen didn't research her condition any further; figuring that her doctor knew best, she went ahead with the hysterectomy. Before this incident, Ellen hadn't had any symptoms of perimenopause. She felt fine for several months after the surgery, but then started waking up in the middle of the night soaked in sweat. She became moody and her hair and skin became drier. Her doctor prescribed 0.625 mg of the estrogenic product Premarin, and her symptoms disappeared.

Several years later, still taking Premarin, she read the Women's Health Initiative study findings, which revealed the risks associated with Premarin. Ellen stopped taking it and tried a homeopathic remedy instead. After six weeks, during which she felt miserable and depressed, she resumed HRT, this time using a bioidentical hormone therapy of estrogen patches and Prometrium (an oral bioidentical progesterone). Ellen knows the bioidentical hormones have made her feel even better, and at sixty-two, she is healthy and active and still enjoys sex. She says her day-to-day quality of life is worth the potential risks (which her research showed to be minimal, given her family history). She also feels it's a much safer alternative than all the drugs she'd have to take to treat the individual symptoms she had, such as depression.

HISTORICAL PERSPECTIVE ON MENOPAUSE

Over the last fifty years, there has been a huge shift in attitudes about menopause in this country. Menopause was first brought to national attention in the 1950s, when Dr. Robert Wilson, a spokesperson for Wyeth-Ayerst, the manufacturer of Premarin, started touting the benefits of their hormone product derived from horse urine. In his book *Feminine Forever*, he tells of a husband who asked him to put his wife on estrogen, reportedly by saying, "She's driving me nuts. She won't fix meals. She picks at me all the time." Then, Wilson says, he took a gun from his pocket and said, "If you don't cure her, I'll kill her" (Wilson 1966, 93).

Dr. Wilson then comments, "I have often been haunted by the thought that except for the tiny stream of estrogen . . . this woman might have died a violent death at the hands of her own husband" (Wilson 1966, 93). Ayerst changed their marketing focus in the 1980s, running an ad that showed a middle-aged woman with a dowager's hump. The focus was now on health and protection from cardiovascular disease and osteoporosis instead of beauty and wifely compliance.

The latest alarm to sound in the world of hormones is the confusing news from the well-publicized Women's Health Initiative study, conducted by the National Institutes of Health. This was a study of horse estrogens and molecularly altered progesterone, which aren't recognized by the body as estrogen and progesterone. The study showed a small increase in strokes, blood clots, heart disease, and breast cancer. These results are not completely surprising, as these substances are foreign to the body and could be expected to have some kind of side effects.

Aggressive marketing, scare tactics, and warnings of dangerous side effects for various treatments add to the confusion and fear that accompany the challenges of menopause. Despite the controversy and social and cultural attitudes, decisions about how to deal with menopause should be made after analyzing your physical symptoms and test results, not out of shame or fear about any course of action. You'll be given objective, quantifiable data about the pros and cons of HRT in chapter 8.

Hysterectomy Alert

Hysterectomy, or the surgical removal of the uterus, has become a very commonly recommended operation both in perimenopause and in the years after menopause. Incredibly, according to the National Uterine Fibroid Foundation (2004) almost 40 percent of the women in the United States have had a hysterectomy by the time they're sixty. This surgery is performed for many reasons, including ovarian cysts, fibroids, uterine prolapse, and excessive bleeding. Many doctors are adamant about the benefits of this surgery, often citing the danger of ovarian cancer. Unfortunately, the hormonal downside to this surgery is rarely explored. Dr. Sarrel published a study showing that a hysterectomy *without removal of the ovaries* resulted in menopause within three months of the surgery for 25 percent of women, and that 60 percent lost ovarian function within three years (Siddle, Sarrel, and Whitehead 1987). These statistics apply to women of *any* age—even those as young as thirty.

Before considering a hysterectomy, it makes sense to try to resolve problems such as excessive bleeding, cysts, and fibroids by correcting imbalances that may have been aggravated by a lack of progesterone. If this fails to resolve the problem, a hysterectomy may be necessary, but given the far-reaching side effects, this should always be a last resort. Even then, if your doctor recommends removing your ovaries along with your uterus, make sure there's a justifiable reason for doing so. In this case, you may need a second (or even third) medical opinion to help clarify your options.

WHAT TO DO ABOUT MENOPAUSE

Because hormone replacement therapy is such a big topic, the next chapter is entirely devoted to this form of treatment for menopausal symptoms. For now, I'll just give you an overview of the two basic schools of thought about menopause. The first says menopause is a natural occurrence that should be experienced naturally, without medication, intervention, or treatment. And though this may be viable for some women, especially the women who have a relatively easy time with the transition, it just isn't true for everyone. Just as natural childbirth works fine, even well, for some women, it doesn't work for everyone, because no two women are the same in terms of physiology, life experience, and even thresholds of pain and discomfort. A contradictory fact is that some women who reject hormone therapy to ease their discomfort during menopause end up taking medications for depression, weight loss, anxiety, pain, and high blood pressure, to name just a few ailments. By giving your body back substances that you used to make, HRT has the potential to address these problems, and depending on which drugs you're taking for menopausal symptoms (and how many), hormones might be a more "natural" path.

One of the first and most famous proponents of natural menopause was the well-known anthropologist Dr. Margaret Mead, who spoke often of her "postmenopausal zest." Such a path is certainly preferable if you are indeed physically able to continue your life as usual. What isn't as widely known, however, is that while Dr. Mead was touting this theory, she was receiving weekly estrogen shots and wasn't postmenopausal at all! She continued to have periods until her sixties (Sheehy 1992).

Up until the Women's Health Initiative results were published, the traditional medical community followed the second school of thought, which was to *always* treat symptoms of hormone imbalance with HRT. Women who went to an ob-gyn with any hormonal complaints at all were encouraged to start on Premarin or Prempro, or at least birth control pills. Many doctors went even further and recommended HRT as a preventive measure against osteoporosis and heart disease even for women who were symptom-free and whose test results were fine. Much of the medical community still advocates this approach, but now they add a warning to take these substances for as short a time as possible—no longer than five years.

Neither of these approaches is universally applicable. The decision to take a prescription drug of any kind needs to be an individual one. But whatever your attitude or situation, please don't base your decision on the theory that since your mother or grandmother didn't need help through menopause, you shouldn't either. Although previous generations generally viewed menopause as an inevitable, natural period of transition, discomfort, or suffering, we live different lives from our mothers and grandmothers. We have our children at a later age, and we work while raising them. More than half of us experience divorce and live as single parents. And, we're doing all of this at an age when our grandmothers were already grandmothers!

Things to Remember

- Every woman's path through perimenopause and menopause is different. Some women have an easy time, and some a terrible time.
- Hormone balance is critical to maintaining a svelte figure as you age. Test your levels of estrogen, thyroid hormones, testosterone, and cortisol to make sure you don't have any imbalances that would sabotage weight-loss efforts. (At this point progesterone is pretty much gone, so there's no need to measure it.)
- Neither the belief that HRT is always necessary or the belief that it is never necessary is correct. Each woman must make this decision based on her own quality of life issues and test data.
- Don't agree to any surgical solution to symptoms of hormone imbalance (such as fibroids or excessive bleeding), including a hysterectomy, until you've researched your individual situation thoroughly. Always get several opinions before scheduling a surgery to make sure this is the best option.

CHAPTER 8

What's Right for You? *Bioidentical Hormone Replacement Therapy*

Lynn's Story

Lynn had always been tall and slender. But at forty-four, she wasn't slender anymore; since she'd turned forty she'd gained 30 pounds and was now up to a distressing 155. Unfortunately, weight gain wasn't the only symptom she'd developed in her forties. She also felt as though she'd lost all control of her emotions. It seemed the slightest thing would make her fly off the handle, and although she felt terrible afterward, she'd often go into another rage an hour later, completely unable to stop herself. She'd started waking up every couple of hours all night long and then usually felt exhausted and befuddled the next day. Her once-shiny auburn hair became dull and dry, and her face appeared drawn and pale.

With all these symptoms making her miserable, Lynn went to her ob-gyn, who started her on Prempro (a combination of Premarin and Provera, forms of estrogen and progesterone that aren't the same as those found naturally in your body). This combination therapy resolved most of her symptoms other than the weight gain, but in her late forties, Lynn began to experience a whole new raft of symptoms, including fatigue and depression. Her doctor started her on an antidepressant, and although this helped with the depression, it left her feeling detached and distracted most of the time. But when the Women's Health Initiative (WHI) findings on Prempro were announced in 2002, Lynn immediately stopped taking the hormones, as they'd been proven to increase the risk of heart disease and breast cancer. Her mother had a heart attack at an early age that left her with seriously compromised health for the rest of her life, so the increase in heart disease risk was enough to change Lynn's mind no matter what the consequences.

However, the sudden cessation of hormones resulted in serious symptoms: Lynn's memory became completely unreliable, her mood swings returned, and she experienced vaginal itching, discomfort, and dryness, the latter resulting in severe pain during sex. Chronic night sweats kept her awake off and on all night, and depression and insomnia began to interfere with her daily life. In despair, Lynn tried to manage her symptoms through a new, rigorous regimen of exercise and diet, but this proved ineffective in relieving her symptoms or affecting her weight gain, which steadily continued. Finally she went to a doctor who tested her hormone levels. The results showed that Lynn was in menopause and also had multiple hormone deficiencies, including low thyroid hormone levels and seriously depleted adrenal function. Her doctor told her that the only way to effectively reduce her symptoms would be with hormone replacement therapy. He said that he understood her reluctance to use Prempro, given the WHI findings, and suggested bioidentical hormones, which might present less risk of heart disease. He wrote a prescription for bioidentical estrogen (Climara patch), progesterone (oral Prometrium), thyroid (Armour Thyroid), and short-term cortisol therapy to rebuild her adrenals, telling her that this would make her feel much better.

Still uneasy about hormones in general after the WHI scare, Lynn was uncomfortable about starting on this new therapy without doing her own research on the risks of heart disease that might be associated with it. On the Internet, she found PubMed, the National Institutes of Health research Web site, and typed in "heart disease and estrogen" and "heart disease and progesterone." The dozen or so research papers on estrogen she read out of the 2,921 available convinced her that not only would estrogen not harm her heart, but that it was actually vital to heart health. She also discovered that most heart disease in women occurs after menopause, when they've run out of estrogen and progesterone (Ballard and Edelberg 2005). In the 520 articles on progesterone and heart disease, there were only a few on bioidentical progesterone and its effects on heart function, but these convinced her that bioidentical progesterone didn't show the same level of risk as Provera (the drug used in the WHI), and it would also effectively reduce the risk of cell proliferation in the uterus and resultant cancer risk caused by estrogen (Rosano, Webb, et al. 2000).

She also learned that transdermal delivery of estrogen (through the skin) more closely mimics the way the ovaries produce and distribute estrogen, so the transdermal product her doctor had prescribed appeared to be the best delivery method. After all of this research, she ended up feeling pretty good—not only about the positive data she found, but also about finally taking charge of her health instead of depending solely on input from others. She started on the estrogen, progesterone, thyroid, and cortisol therapy, and after taking a month or two to arrive at the right dosage of each, she felt like her old self again. The first things she noticed were that her hot flashes and all other symptoms of low estrogen resolved, and that she had regained her sense of humor and formerly calm disposition. Then she felt her energy coming back and, like a miracle, she finally started to lose weight.

SOME BACKGROUND ON HRT

If you're starting to feel the effects of dropping hormone levels and are dreading the changes to come, stop fearing and start learning, as Lynn did. This is your opportunity to figure out what your body is going through and design a plan to maintain your health and even your youthfulness. We are not a generation that has taken anything lying down; we were raised to question and analyze, and to chart our own path. Where better to apply this approach than to the aging process? There is truly no need to suffer through "the change of life." And if your research, test results, and symptoms all point to HRT, then you should by all means consider this option.

The Women's Health Initiative Study

After years and years of doctors prescribing oral Premarin, estrogens derived from horse urine, evidence started mounting that it was causing an increase in uterine and breast cancer. To counter the proliferative effects of this nonhuman estrogen and reduce the risk of uterine cancer, Provera (which is similar but not identical to progesterone, the body's natural balance for estrogen) was added to the Premarin, creating the drug Prempro. As use of this molecularly altered form of progesterone grew, so did the incidence of breast cancer, which was already increased slightly by the use of Premarin. Provera also reversed the positive effects that Premarin had on cardiovascular health when the two were used in combination, and had negative effects on bone density when used alone as a contraceptive.

In response to this growing concern, in 1991 the National Institutes of Health began the Women's Health Initiative (WHI), a series of large clinical trials studying Provera and Premarin. These studies were halted prematurely in 2002, when findings suggested that there were possible health risks associated with using horse estrogen and altered progesterone, and that they caused a slight increase in strokes, blood clots, heart disease, and breast cancer.

Unfortunately, when the findings from the WHI were published, the media failed to clarify the distinction between the hormone products tested and bioidentical hormones. It was never made clear that actual bioidentical women's hormones weren't being tested in the WHI. The only word publicized was "hormones," so the medical community understandably responded by taking most of their patients off all hormones. Although this has been a major setback to hormone use

... general, one positive outcome of this study is that a lot of attention has been focused on this issue. The word is finally starting to get out, thanks to many committed women, including the efforts of celebrity advocates like Suzanne Somers, that not only does standard HRT use hormones unnatural to the body, but also that these synthetic hormones have negative side effects. So please keep in mind that the following discussions of hormone replacement options refer *only* to natural, bioidentical hormones.

What Are Bioidentical Hormones?

Bioidentical hormones are identical in every way to the hormones produced in our bodies. The distinction between these bioidentical hormones and the hormone products that have been widely marketed in the past is extremely important to understand. If it seems counterintuitive to use hormones in other forms than those that are made in our bodies and that have worked so well for most of our lives, it will be helpful for you to learn a little bit about the way the pharmaceutical industry works.

Since U.S. patent law prevents companies from patenting molecules that naturally occur in the human body, to get patent protection pharmaceutical companies have developed products that are made of substances not found in our bodies. This makes a great deal of business sense, as a patent protects a product from competition for up to twenty years. The patented hormone products that have been widely prescribed for the last forty years are oral estrogen (Premarin) and progesterone (Provera). Premarin is derived from horses (the name, believe it or not, comes from "pregnant mare's urine"), and Provera is a chemically altered form of progesterone; both are therefore patentable. While they may make business sense, these products don't make much sense for us women. In fact, they don't even register as hormones in blood tests! But when you supplement bioidentical hormones, which are generally made from soy or yam extracts and then altered to have the same molecular structure as the hormones made by your own body, they'll show up as estrogen and progesterone in lab tests. This allows you to monitor your levels and balance the relationship between them.

There haven't been any large clinical studies of bioidentical hormones, and the reason is clear: Without patents to protect them from competition, there's no economic incentive for pharmaceutical companies to underwrite extensive studies. Several small studies have been done on bioidentical hormones; however, there's no conclusive safety or efficacy data to date. But what is available is a steadily growing body of research that shows the ability of estrogen and progesterone to resolve symptoms and have positive effects on a variety of diseases and conditions associated with aging, including osteoporosis, heart disease, and the function of the brain, vagina, and bladder. Until we have data on the effects of bioidentical HRT, a commonsense approach suggests using substances that are exactly the same as those in the body to replace what's lost as we age, in a pattern as close to the body's natural biological rhythms as possible. With this approach, the risks should be far lower than when foreign substances are introduced in a manner foreign to the body.

HORMONE REPLACEMENT THERAPY OPTIONS

The surprising findings of the WHI shocked most doctors into one of two responses: immobility, causing them to leave their patients on their current *non*bioidentical therapy (with possibly a few more restrictions), or panic, causing them to take all their patients off HRT altogether. The current "restricted" HRT path now recommended by doctors who prescribe Prempro or Premarin is focused on low-dose, short-term treatment of symptoms as women transition into menopause (generally over eighteen to twenty-four months). The stated goals of this approach are to relieve menopausal symptoms caused by estrogen deficiency, prevent and treat osteoporosis, protect against cardiovascular disease, delay symptoms of Alzheimer's disease, and possibly protect against colon cancer. This is somewhat confusing, however, since short-term therapy wouldn't affect long-term conditions like heart disease, osteoporosis, and cognitive decline.

Whereas Prempro and Premarin are generally prescribed in a one-size-fits-all fashion, many doctors who work with bioidentical hormone replacement tend to look at a more individualized picture. They generally agree on replacing hormones for women who are experiencing unpleasant symptoms, whose hormone levels are low in lab tests, or who have quantifiable risk factors, such as a family or personal history of heart disease, osteoporosis, or Alzheimer's disease. These doctors try to replace hormones in as close to the body's normal rhythm as possible, and they track levels with lab tests to make sure estrogen and progesterone are in balance.

The goal is to try to replicate as closely as possible what goes on naturally in the human body, in terms of molecular structure, timing, quantities, and route of delivery.

After much research, we believe that estradiol is the only form of estrogen that women should replace. Estradiol is the form of estrogen that naturally does all the work to keep our bodies and minds young and functioning well until menopause. Some doctors recommend estriol or even estrone for hormone replacement. However, your body can make estrone and estriol from estradiol so there's no reason to add more, particularly since too much estrone has negative consequences, such as high blood sugar, diabetes, early heart attacks, or strokes. Estriol is only present in minute amounts except during pregnancy, and it hasn't been shown to be as protective of the brain, bones, heart, or other organs as estradiol. Furthermore, it's not currently approved for human use in the United States and can be only obtained through compound pharmacies.

Replicating your body's natural hormonal rhythms also means supplementing with bioidentical progesterone whenever estrogen is replaced. Whenever this book suggests using HRT, I mean supplementing both estrogen *and* progesterone. I believe strongly that estrogen should never be used without progesterone.

The Importance of Progesterone in HRT

The current standard-of-care approach is that it's not necessary to supplement progesterone if you don't have a uterus. This may be safe, but there are no large clinical studies that demonstrate that it's safe and effective to supplement estrogen without progesterone. Doctors are adamant that women take progesterone as long as they have a uterus, but your breasts and other body parts should also be considered along with your uterus. Progesterone receptors are found throughout the body (including in the brain, breasts, and vagina) and occur in most of the same places where estrogen receptors are found. Cell proliferation can be a problem in any of these areas when estrogen is present and not balanced by progesterone.

The only time women naturally have high levels of estrogen is during our youth, when we always have significant amounts of progesterone as well. Supplementing progesterone to mimic the natural cycle is unappealing for some women after menopause, because adding progesterone for two weeks out of the month results in a continuation of periods. This occurs because when progesterone replacement stops on day twenty-eight, it causes the uterine lining to begin breaking down, and a few days later it is shed from the uterus. To avoid this, many doctors give menopausal women continuous progesterone therapy all month long. This prevents your monthly periods because continual progesterone maintains the uterine lining. It would be nice not to have periods, but your body is given a break from progesterone for two weeks out of the month for a reason: Progesterone blocks the effects and benefits of estrogen even as it protects against excessive cell proliferation, so if given continuously, progesterone can potentially negate some of the substantial benefits of estrogen.

There's also some thought that it may be safe to add progesterone only every couple of months instead of every month, to shed the uterine lining and prevent the overgrowth that can cause dysplasia or other abnormal cell growth. This would reduce the number of menstrual periods to one every couple of months, but it hasn't been clinically studied, so its safety is unknown. For the time being, the safest course of action is to add progesterone for the last two weeks of every cycle to replicate your body's natural rhythm. When you think of how well this works for us while we're still reproductively viable, it makes sense.

Many women try progesterone-only replacement (without estrogen) after seeing marketing materials touting its benefits. But as discussed in earlier chapters, even though progesterone is important, it's only effective if you have enough estrogen to make progesterone receptors. Unless you're using progesterone to balance your own high estrogen levels, you should consider combining it with estrogen replacement.

Sorting Out the Risks and Benefits of HRT

When you start your research on HRT, you'll see almost immediately that estrogen replacement therapy has been quite controversial and has generated a great deal of confusion, fear, and emotion. In recent years, the risks of hormone replacement with *non*bioidentical hormones have been well publicized. Some of these negative side effects appear to be related to the chemical alteration of these substances and haven't been proven to apply to the hormones we make in our bodies. Small-scale studies on the use of bioidentical hormones for specific conditions have

It Could Be Worse

Hormone replacement options are becoming increasingly fine-tuned and sophisticated. We've come a long way from eighteenth-century Europe (thank goodness!), when menopause treatment included consuming raw eggs and/or powdered donkey penis, followed by being bled by leeches to rid the body of toxins. By the 1900s in Paris, when the link between hot flashes and ovarian function had been discovered, women were prescribed sandwiches of sheep's ovaries in unleavened bread to help with symptoms, and shortly after this, ovarian extracts started to be given by injection (Richardson 1973).

demonstrated that they don't seem to present the same risks. If you compare bioidentical hormone therapy to other pharmaceutical drug treatments, you'd be hard-pressed to find another treatment that has such incredible, proven, long-term success coupled with so few side effects. This makes sense because, in effect, these hormones have been tested in humans as long as human beings have existed. Unfortunately, without the large, long-term clinical studies on bioidentical hormones that would give us definitive information, the best course of action isn't clear. Even more unfortunate is the fact that these studies probably won't be done anytime soon.

It's also important to note that, although sensationalized, the risk statistics associated with the nonbioidentical hormones studied in the WHI weren't overly negative. The average risk per woman was approximately a 0.1 percent increase per year for breast cancer or heart attack. Unfortunately, the media stated the findings as percentages of *relative risk*, saying that the increase in breast cancer was 26 percent, coronary heart disease 29 percent, stroke 41 percent, and pulmonary embolism 213 percent. However, when the figures are given in terms of *absolute risk*, they represent eight additional cases of breast cancer, seven heart attacks, eight strokes, and eight pulmonary embolisms for every ten thousand women. And although this didn't receive the same sort of attention, the study actually showed several types of risk reduction: six fewer colorectal cancers and five fewer hip fractures per ten thousand women (Sturdee 2004). Also, there was no difference between the groups in terms of mortality. The risk statistics associated with HRT are much lower than those of many other drugs on the market, many of them with therapeutic effects that are far less wide-ranging.

Another problem is that the WHI studied women with an average age of sixty-four—much older than the average hormone user. Women generally start hormone therapy around the time of menopause, when their symptoms get dramatically worse. The benefits of HRT appear to decrease the longer women wait to start treatment. Studies show that when women start hormone therapy soon after menopause, they reduce their risk of coronary heart disease by 30 percent (Grodstein, Manson, and Stampfer 2006). This is possibly because estrogen protects their blood vessels, keeping them smooth and free of plaque. But when women go without estrogen for a long period of time, they tend to develop atherosclerosis. Replacing estrogen once atherosclerosis is a factor may cause problems, because it increases the tendency to clot and thus increases the risk of a heart attack.

Bernadine Healy, MD, director of the National Institutes of Health during the WHI, has said that the average age of women studied was a valid explanation for the negative results. She reassured women who were taking Premarin not to worry, since it "had no net benefit but also no net harm." Furthermore, she endorsed the use of hormones for women who needed them, saying "the risk of HRT is tiny" (Healy 2004).

The risks associated with bioidentical hormones appear to be even less for a couple of reasons. Horse estrogens add a slight risk for breast cancer, but when chemically altered progesterone is added, the risk increases to the numbers mentioned above. In several studies, estrogen alone was shown to have positive effects on heart health but, again, this benefit was lost when chemically altered progesterone was added (Sitruk-Ware 2000). Additionally, animal studies have shown that bioidentical progesterone may have the advantage of not reducing estrogen's ability to inhibit atherosclerosis, as chemically altered progesterone does (Adams et al. 1990). These animal studies suggest that the chemical alteration of the progesterone is creating the negative effect, rather than the progesterone itself.

RISKS ASSOCIATED WITH HRT

The following statistics on risk factors for various conditions were determined by studies of *non*bioidentical hormones, but they may also apply to bioidentical hormones.

Breast cancer: Research suggests an increased risk of breast cancer of approximately 1 percent with estrogen use (Schairer et al. 2000), but not all the evidence supports this finding (Gapstur, Morrow, and Sellers 1999). The risk appears to be related to duration of use, with longer-term users being more affected (Lando, Heck, and Brett 1999). Current opinion is that HRT taken for less than five years doesn't significantly increase the risk of breast cancer, but studies have shown a small increased risk after five years of use.

Blood clots: HRT has been shown to cause a small increase in risk of blood clots (Miller, Chan, and Nelson 2002). This should be investigated further if you have a personal or family history of blood clots. There is some evidence that transdermal estrogen (delivered through the skin) may not cause the same increased risk (Tikkanen 1996).

Heart disease: Recent studies such as HERS (the Heart and Estrogen-Progestin Replacement Study) and the WHI suggest that certain types of HRT may cause a small increased risk for heart disease. The factors that appear to influence whether estrogen replacement creates increased risk for a particular woman are the method of administration, the dose of estrogen, whether chemically altered progesterone is used with the estrogen, the age of the woman, and if she had coronary artery disease before starting HRT. Women who start replacement shortly after menopause, before heart disease has had time to develop, don't appear to have increased risk.

Endometrial cancer: Estrogen-only therapy given to women who still have a uterus increases their risk of endometrial hyperplasia (thickening of the lining of the uterus), and eventually increases their risk of endometrial cancer. Using progesterone for ten to fourteen days per month reduces the risk but doesn't completely eliminate it. If taken for more than five years, this sequential HRT dosing does increase the risk of endometrial cancer by a small amount, but it appears that there's no increased risk when estrogen is combined with daily progesterone.

BENEFITS ASSOCIATED WITH HRT

The ability of estrogen (coupled with progesterone for balance) to affect the course of aging is enormous. It prevents disease and promotes quality of life—from strength and endurance to strong bones to mental acuity to heart health to happiness and positive outlook (and let's not forget great skin and hair!). During our reproductive years, when our hormone levels are high, we are astonishingly resistant to aging. We can abuse ourselves through bad diet, lack of exercise, not enough sleep, and numerous other ways and still be remarkably healthy. We don't get heart attacks or strokes, and our immune function is prodigious. For most of us, it's only when we enter perimenopause that we start to see greatly increased health problems.

It's important to study and evaluate the risks associated with any potential hormone replacement therapy, but we can't lose sight of the substantial benefits of supplementing estrogen and progesterone. The FDA has studied and approved estrogen for the treatment of hot flashes, vaginal dryness, and osteoporosis, and many other benefits of estrogen have been well studied and quantified.

Hot flashes: Hot flashes and night sweats are almost always cured by estrogen replacement. In fact, these symptoms are often used as a barometer to see if HRT dosing is correct; if you start having them again, your estrogen dose is too low.

Vaginal and urinary tract changes: Both the bladder and the vagina respond very well to HRT. Symptoms of low estrogen such as burning, itching, painful intercourse, frequent vaginal and bladder infections, and urinary incontinence resolve quickly. Estrogen increases blood flow, thickens the walls of the vagina and bladder, and increases lubrication, critical for comfortable and enjoyable sexual intercourse.

Mood swings: Many clinical studies have proven that HRT has a marked effect on the irritability, depression, and mood swings that often appear during perimenopause and menopause (Heinrich and Wolf 2005). There's also evidence that depression is a result of fluctuating estrogen rather than low estrogen (Good, Day, and Muir 1999). This is why there's an increased incidence of psychological symptoms and depression in women between the ages of forty-five and forty-nine, when estrogen levels are generally very erratic.

Bone health: Combined estrogen and progesterone therapy has been found to decrease bone loss and promote new bone growth (Prior 1990). When we lose our estrogen supply, bone density typically decreases by about 2 percent per year in the spine and 1 percent per year in the hip, although it can be as high as 10 percent in the spine and 5 percent in the hip for women predisposed to osteoporosis. Women lose approximately 50 percent of their skeleton by age seventy, while men lose only 25 percent by age ninety.

Brain function: HRT increases memory and cognitive abilities and potentially reduces risk of Alzheimer's disease. Alzheimer's causes nerve cells to lose connections with neighboring cells and develop abnormal proteins that interfere with normal cognitive functioning. A study done at Leisure World Laguna Hills, a retirement community in California, showed that women who took estrogen were 35 percent less likely to develop Alzheimer's, with the greatest risk reduction in those who used estrogen for the longest period of time at the highest doses (Paganini-Hill and Henderson 1996). In fact, a 2001 study reported significant benefits after just four weeks of HRT with estrogen patches (Asthana et al. 2001). Several other studies have demonstrated that HRT also decreases risk for dementia by approximately 50 percent (Sano 2000). However, not all studies have demonstrated estrogen to be protective for Alzheimer's, and more research is needed to confirm these findings.

Heart benefits: Studies have shown that estrogen replacement has beneficial effects on lipid metabolism, which include reducing "bad" LDL cholesterol and increasing "good" HDL cholesterol (Nanda et al. 2003). If you have a family history of heart disease, high blood pressure, high cholesterol, diabetes, or an enlarged heart, you may benefit from HRT.

Skin protection and rejuvenation: Estrogen has an enormous effect on your skin. It plays a role in the way fat is distributed under the skin. This fat provides firmness to the skin and keeps it plumped up and youthful. Loss of estrogen also causes lower collagen levels, and collagen is responsible for your skin's firmness and elasticity. Approximately 30 percent of skin collagen is lost in the first five years after menopause. Estrogen also is responsible for maintenance of skin thickness and water retention, so when levels drop, skin gets dry and flaky. Of course, having younger-looking skin isn't a reason to start HRT, but it's a side effect most of us don't mind.

IS HORMONE REPLACEMENT THERAPY RIGHT FOR YOU?

The question of whether to replace hormones wouldn't have occurred to many women prior to the twentieth century; not only was this not an option, most women weren't even fortunate enough to live very long beyond their childbearing years. But women can now expect to live to eighty-five or older, so we need to think about how to live these additional years (which could be one-third to one-half of our life) in good spirits and good health. This means we need to think about how we can support our aging endocrine systems, and bioidentical hormone replacement is one of the most valuable tools available to accomplish this.

Whether to use HRT is a decision each woman must make for herself, but before you decide, consider not just your symptoms and well-being, but also other, less obvious health changes. To detect these potential health conditions, you need to have a complete physical: How are your cholesterol levels and your blood pressure? Are you insulin resistant? Have you had your bone density measured? You may have conditions that will undermine your future health but can be prevented, or corrected and reversed, by starting hormone therapy early. One of the most obvious and measurable of these is osteoporosis. Measuring the status of your bones with a DEXA scan (dual energy X-ray absorptiometry)—considered to be the most reliable test currently available—allows you to determine whether you have the beginnings of bone loss and whether you're at risk for serious osteoporosis. If you are, HRT may make sense for you, as it's impossible to reverse lost height or fractures in your vertebrae once they've occurred. On the other hand, it's also important to look at your family history for risk factors, as you did in chapter 2, before you blithely start on hormone replacement.

If you don't have any obvious risk factors for osteoporosis, cardiovascular disease, or Alzheimer's disease and your menopausal symptoms (such as hot flashes and insomnia) aren't significant or long-lasting, you may have no real need for HRT. There are, however, certain circumstances that most doctors agree indicate the need for HRT (and almost always at higher dosing levels). If you have an autoimmune disorder, or if you had premature ovarian failure or a hysterectomy before you were menopausal, you'll most likely benefit greatly from HRT. On the other hand, some conditions preclude HRT, such as unexplained vaginal bleeding, pregnancy, active thrombosis or thrombophlebitis, endometrial adenocarcinoma, estrogen-dependent tumors, and active liver disease. However, since most of us don't fall into either of these two groups, the decision isn't clear-cut for most women.

EXERCISE: Assessing Your Potential Risks and Benefits from HRT

Without conclusive evidence as to the safety of bioidentical hormone therapy, whether to take hormones becomes an individual decision. Before deciding, sit down and review your personal and family health history and all of the exercises that you've completed while working through this book. Beyond analyzing all of that information, it's also important that you answer the following questions and consider the implications of your answers before making a decision whether to start HRT. Provide full details on any that you answer yes to. It will be important to share this information with your doctor.

1. Have any of your female relatives had breast cancer? If so, at what age? Was the cancer estrogen-positive?

____

____

____

2. Have any of your female relatives had uterine cancer?

____

____

____

3. Do any of your family members have osteoporosis?

____

____

____

4. When did your mother enter menopause? Did she have a difficult experience? (If your mother had a hysterectomy, it's important that you and your doctor know why.)

____

____

____

5. Is there a history of high blood pressure or heart disease in your family?

____

____

____

6. Have any of your female relatives had long-term, debilitating PMS?

____

____

____

7. Have any of your relatives had dementia or Alzheimer's disease?

____

____

____

Questions 1 and 2 indicate possible risk factors for HRT. If you have a personal or family history of breast or uterine cancer, you should explore this issue further with your doctor before proceeding with HRT. Questions 3 through 7 can indicate a potential for HRT to be beneficial for you; if you answer yes to any of these questions, it could indicate a predisposition for conditions and diseases related to hormone deficiency.

EXERCISE: Evaluating How HRT May Improve Your Quality of Life

Evaluating medical and health risks is a crucial part of any decision about whether to use HRT, but there are other important aspects of your life that may be impacted by your hormonal status and how you decide to proceed. Don't overlook thinking about your quality of life and the health of your relationships. Ask yourself the following questions and, in your journal, answer them as honestly as you can:

- Just how uncomfortable or miserable are you?
- Are your symptoms affecting your ability to function in everyday life?
- Are your relationships (with your spouse, kids, friends, or family) starting to suffer because of your symptoms?

Think about all of the ramifications of your answers, then talk to your friends (always a critical element in the equation for us women) to find out what experiences they've had with, or without, hormone replacement.

FDA-Approved and Compound Pharmacy Products

If you've decided to try HRT, deciding what drugs to use is just as important as deciding whether to use them or not, as they can dramatically affect the success of your therapy. There are currently two general types of prescription bioidentical hormones for HRT on the market: FDA-approved drugs manufactured by pharmaceutical companies, and drugs made by compound pharmacies, which are not FDA-approved. The FDA-approved estradiol products (including patches, cream, pills, or gel) and progesterone products (pills or vaginal gel) are all of excellent quality. They're manufactured under rigorous FDA guidelines just like any other pharmaceutical product. The following are the most commonly prescribed products. (See appendix B for data on the blood levels of estrogen and progesterone these products generate in the body.)

- Estrogen products:
    - **Patches:** Vivelle-Dot, Climara, Alora, Esclim, and Estraderm. These come in varying strengths—0.025, 0.0375, 0.05,

0.06, 0.075, and 0.1 mg. Manufacturers recommend these be changed weekly or biweekly, depending on the product, but many women find that they run out sooner (as evidenced by the return of obvious symptoms such as hot flashes and headaches) and need to be changed more often.

- **Topical gel:** EstroGel—daily (0.75 mg pump)
- **Topical cream:** Estrasorb—daily (0.025 mg per packet)
- **Oral:** Estrace—daily (0.05, 1, and 2 mg)

- Progesterone products:
  - **Oral:** Prometrium—daily (100 and 200 mg)
  - **Intravaginal gel:** Prochieve or Crinone—every other day (4 or 8 percent)

Compounded drugs must be purchased through specialized *compounding pharmacies*—pharmacies that have the capability to make drugs out of bulk chemicals. These drugs aren't approved by the FDA, but they're legally sold under a special allowance by the FDA primarily to accommodate individualized dosing regimens. They aren't manufactured under FDA guidelines and can vary widely in effect. The raw materials used in compounded drugs aren't required to be tested for efficacy, so it's common that one month's prescription of compounded hormones may be very strong and provide excellent symptom resolution, and the next month's prescription will have virtually no effect at all. This is confusing to most women and their doctors, who believe that if the drug requires a prescription, the quality is ensured.

The pharmacies that compound these drugs are generally very reputable and skilled at compounding (mixing) ingredients, but if the raw material they start with has limited efficacy, then the final drug will as well. In 2001, the FDA analyzed product samples from twelve compounding pharmacies and found that 34 percent of them failed one or more standard quality tests, including potency tests, and all contained less of the active ingredient than expected. In contrast, the testing failure rate for FDA-approved drug therapies is less than 2 percent (American College of Obstetricians and Gynecologists 2005).

I used compounded drugs for years before I discovered the FDA-approved estrogen patches, but I had to get my levels of estrogen and progesterone measured almost every month just to manage the dosing. One month I would have a robust estrogen level of 300 pg/ml, and the next it would be down to 60 pg/ml. I would adjust my dose up according to the test results (and how I felt), but this resulted in constantly fluctuating hormone levels, which caused symptoms of hormone imbalance.

The positive side to compound drugs is that you *can* have a very individualized dosing protocol—you and your doctor can change levels and fine-tune your dosage. However, your doctor will generally want you to measure your hormone levels regularly so you can adjust your dose to accommodate varying product strength. Estradiol, estriol, and progesterone from compounding pharmacies come in oral, sublingual cream, or suppository form.

How Much Estrogen and Progesterone Should You Take?

There are many schools of thought on dosing levels for hormone replacement. In the aftermath of WHI, many doctors who prescribe either bioidentical or nonbioidentical hormones now advocate using the lowest levels of estrogen and progesterone possible. However, many women need higher levels to resolve their symptoms and achieve good health. Maybe they always had higher levels, so that's what their bodies are used to, or maybe they have extremely severe symptoms and need higher amounts to counteract them. The premise behind higher levels of hormones is that estrogen and progesterone are not just sex or reproductive hormones, they're also essential for many critical functions, such as memory, muscle strength, hearing, cognition, and vision. Without these hormones, a woman's body begins to age and lose functionality. Most advocates of higher dosing levels recommend staying on hormones for the rest of your life to achieve continuous benefits and prevent disease.

To find your optimal dosing level, your doctor may decide to simply adjust doses of estrogen and progesterone until you find relief from your symptoms, taking into consideration your history and symptoms. Many doctors will have a standard dose that they start their patients on: for patch products, between 0.025 and 0.1 mg, or for oral products, between 0.05 and 2.50 mg (once or twice a day). They'll adjust this initial dose up or down, depending on the woman's response.

One way to begin your dosing protocol is to look at the average levels of estrogen and progesterone in the graph in chapter 1. The graph will give you an idea of the range your body is most likely used to. As the graph indicates, most women don't go much below 80 pg/ml in estrogen levels at their lowest monthly point. This is consistent with the findings of Dr. Elizabeth Vliet, an HRT pioneer: that her patients feel best when they keep their estrogen levels over 90 to 100 pg/ml (Vliet 1995). The graph also shows that estrogen levels are higher in the second half of the menstrual cycle. This is something you'll want to keep in mind if you end up with symptoms of high progesterone and low estrogen during this time (just as you may have in perimenopause). If this happens, you may want to consider using a slightly higher dose of estrogen during the two weeks you're supplementing progesterone.

What I Learned

It took a lot of trial and error to arrive at my current dosing regimen, which has relieved all my symptoms (and even then, I had to add thyroid and cortisol replacement to become completely symptom-free). I started out on a very high-dose regimen of compounded estrogen and progesterone creams that was becoming popular in Santa Barbara several years ago. The goal of this approach was to restore the hormonal rhythms and levels of youth.

It was a complex dosing protocol that changed doses every day in an attempt to replicate the body's natural production of both estrogen and progesterone, creating two peaks of estrogen (on days thirteen and twenty-one) and a peak of progesterone (on day twenty-one). I was willing to take the risk of using very high levels of estrogen and progesterone, since the alternative of progressing multiple sclerosis left me barely able to function. Unfortunately, although I found significant relief with this protocol (as I would have with any protocol that augmented my nonexistent levels of both hormones), the widely fluctuating levels, along with the variable quality of the compounded estrogen and progesterone, caused continued symptoms of hormone imbalance. Only when I did further research did I find that one of the keys to how bad your symptoms get is how greatly your hormone levels fluctuate. If they swing rapidly and drastically, you'll feel much worse than if they remain stable and balanced, even if the overall levels are lower.

While using this complicated dosing regimen, I faithfully tested my estrogen and progesterone levels twice a month (on day thirteen, when I was attempting to mimic ovulation, and on day twenty-one, on my progesterone peak). I kept my hormone levels very high, but I feel much better now on a lower, stable dose. The symptoms of imbalance went away when I started to use transdermal time-release estrogen patches and intravaginal time-release progesterone gel, keeping my levels very consistent and steady.

Through this process of trial and error, I've learned that HRT is a very individual thing—one size most definitely *does not* fit all. I've been involved with many great doctors who are on the cutting edge of hormone replacement and have spoken to numerous women on HRT, and one thing that consistently stands out is that few women respond in exactly the same way to the same dose. Don't get discouraged if it takes you a couple of months to arrive at the right dose of estrogen or progesterone (or even thyroid or cortisol, if your individual condition warrants it).

What to Do Before You Start HRT

It's always better to err on the side of caution when considering any drug regimen, so if you've decided that your symptoms or health risks merit HRT, please work with your doctor to undergo all of the following tests and evaluations before you start. It's important that you be tested for levels of estrogen, progesterone, testosterone, thyroid hormones, and cortisol. (Details on these lab tests appear in chapters 4 through 6.) In addition to having your hormone levels tested, have a gynecological checkup, a comprehensive metabolic profile, and evaluations for heart

Oral, Transdermal, Intravaginal . . . What Delivery Method Should You Use?

Hormones can be delivered in several different ways: orally; through a patch on the skin; using a cream or gel rubbed into the skin; with an intrauterine device; via a suppository, vaginal ring, or vaginal gel; or, infrequently, by injection. The delivery method may depend on the symptoms you're treating. For instance, a vaginal estrogen ring or cream delivers estrogen directly to the vagina and can ease vaginal dryness, urinary leakage, or vaginal or urinary infections, but it generally won't relieve hot flashes and most other symptoms.

Estrogen taken orally goes directly to the liver, where much of it is processed and broken down, creating substances called *metabolites*. Oral doses must be much higher to get enough estrogen through the liver and provide a high enough blood level to be effective, and there's a downside to this: At least half of any oral estrogen you take is converted to estrone metabolites, and high levels of estrone are linked to certain cancers and heart disease. In light of this, estrogen is optimally replaced by transdermal delivery (a patch, or gel or cream rubbed into the skin). Transdermal medicine is absorbed at a much higher level than oral medicine, which must first be broken down in the liver, so transdermal doses can generally be lower than oral doses of the same medicine. (It's a little scary to think of everything we've put on our skin over our lifetimes. We sometimes forget that the skin is just one massive organ and that most substances we put on it, including potentially toxic substances like fingernail polish remover and cleaning products, get absorbed very effectively.)

Using estrogen patches makes a lot of sense, as the estrogen is released very slowly, closely mimicking the body's own production. Creams and gels are also viable alternatives, but women without much body fat generally get too much variation in their levels when they use these forms, since they have insufficient fat to store the estrogen for slow release. This is in part because hormones are *lipophilic*, or fat loving, so they'll migrate to adipose tissue, where they're stored and released slowly.

Progesterone can be delivered orally, vaginally, or through a cream rubbed into the skin. Either vaginal or transdermal delivery is optimal, so it doesn't first go to the liver for processing, creating metabolites. Vaginal delivery of the progesterone products Prochieve and Crinone has proven to provide higher, less variable blood levels than oral progesterone (Levine and Watson 2000).

disease and bone health. You should also review your personal and family health history and share any relevant information with your doctor if you haven't already done so.

HORMONE LEVELS

It's a good idea to keep track of all your lab reports in one place for easy reference. Chapter 4 includes a handy form for recording these results, which you can photocopy and add to your journal. When recording your results, note whether any of your levels were out of range, indicating an excess or deficiency, to help you decide whether you should consider HRT.

GYNECOLOGICAL CHECKUP

A thorough gynecological checkup should include a Pap smear, breast exam, and mammogram. If you're concerned about the radiation risks associated with mammograms, you might consider a breast ultrasound, but be aware that this procedure is relatively costly and still not covered by most insurance plans. You should also have a pelvic ultrasound to determine the thickness of your uterine lining. It's important to make sure the lining isn't thicker than it should be and that you don't have any cysts, fibroids, or other conditions that might be a cause for concern and additional evaluation. If your checkup or mammogram shows any unusual results, note these in your journal and follow up with your doctor to get to the bottom of what's going on.

HEART DISEASE EVALUATION

The three tests described below can help indicate your risk of heart disease. Determining your waist-to-hip ratio is easy to do at home, but you'll need lab tests to determine any insulin resistance or problematic levels of cholesterol or triglycerides. Follow your doctor's directions for each test, and record the results of each test in your journal. Always request copies of any lab results from your doctor for your own permanent health file. Your doctor will alert you to any problems these tests uncover, but you should also review the results yourself to see where you fall in the reference range. If you fall within the "normal" range but are near the top or bottom, you'll want to keep an eye on potentially problematic levels. If this is the case, talk with your doctor to see if it's advisable to retest at some point in the future to make sure your levels are still okay. If any of your results indicate cause for concern, consult with your doctor to figure out how to address the situation.

Waist-to-hip ratio: This test measures where your fat is located and how much you have. If you store your fat in your upper body, you have what's commonly called an "apple" body type. If you have the "pear" body type, your fat is stored in your hips and thighs. The apple body type indicates a greater risk for heart disease and diabetes. To get your waist-to-hip ratio, measure your hips at their widest point and your waist at its narrowest point. Divide your waist measurement by your hip measurement. If the result is greater than 0.8, you have an apple shape and should be concerned about risk factors for heart disease and diabetes.

Insulin resistance: Insulin resistance indicates risk for both diabetes and heart disease. Several blood tests will shed light on this risk factor: fasting glucose, fasting insulin, and glucose tolerance (with insulin).

Lipid profile test: This test measures your blood levels of cholesterol (HDL and LDL) and triglycerides. HDL, or "good" cholesterol, takes plaque away from artery walls to the liver for excretion, increases blood flow in the body, and decreases the formation of blood clots. It also helps to remove LDL, or "bad" cholesterol, from your system. The ratio of total cholesterol to HDL cholesterol is useful in predicting atherosclerosis: the higher the ratio, the greater risk of heart attack. The average ratio is about 4.5, with 2 or 3 being optimal. High triglyceride levels have been linked to coronary artery disease in some people. High levels may also be a consequence of other diseases, such as untreated diabetes mellitus. This test should be done while fasting to get the most accurate results.

OTHER IMPORTANT TESTS

Again, record the results of the tests below in your journal; or you might photocopy lengthy test reports and insert them in your journal. If any results show cause for concern, be sure to follow up with your doctor to figure out what's going on and how to address the situation.

Comprehensive metabolic profile: This blood test looks at kidney function, liver function, electrolytes, proteins, glucose, and calcium. It will screen for any metabolic problems that could be causing your symptoms or health conditions.

Bone health evaluation: The DEXA scan (dual energy X-ray absorptiometry), which measures bone density at the hip and spine, is thought to be the most accurate bone density test currently available.

FINDING AND WORKING WITH YOUR DOCTOR

Half the challenge of ensuring proper hormone balance is finding the right doctor. It's essential that you find a doctor who's willing to work with you to detect and treat any hormonal deficiencies affecting your current health or quality of life, as well as any conditions that could affect your future health, such as heart disease or osteoporosis. You'll need proper testing and evaluation over a period of time, and because the process needs to be interactive, you should consider your doctor your partner. You need to be able to count on getting lab results back quickly, and you need to be able to reach your doctor to discuss the results. When you start on HRT, you'll most likely need to adjust your dosing levels in the first few months, so it's essential that the communication channels be open. Women who discontinue HRT often do so because of side effects caused by problems with the initial dose, and it's common to have to try several different dosing protocols to figure out what's optimal for you. Therefore, your success may be dependent on good communication with your doctor and frequent contact during this early phase. Fortunately, many women are happy with the first regimen they try.

It's important to find a doctor who not only has training and experience in bioidentical hormones, but who is also open to listening to you and taking into consideration your goals and needs. You deserve a doctor who will spend the time required to analyze your entire situation. This means looking at your personal and family health history, taking the time to go through all of your symptoms, and treating you as a whole person, rather than just isolated body parts. If your doctor sees your vagina as somehow unrelated to the rest of your body and recommends an estrogen vaginal ring to treat your severe symptoms of vaginal dryness but ignores all the other symptoms you have (such as hot flashes, insomnia, and depression), keep looking until you find someone who recognizes that extreme vaginal dryness is only the tip of the iceberg and should be investigated further.

It was important for me to find someone who would work with me to create an HRT protocol that would resolve all my symptoms. This ultimately involved "off-label" usage of FDA-approved products, meaning using FDA products at different dosing levels than the FDA has approved. In my case, this meant using two estrogen patches instead of one. To work effectively with my doctor, I had to make her confident that I would take personal and financial responsibility for checking my hormone levels. This ensured that my hormone levels were in the appropriate range and that my estrogen was effectively balanced by adequate progesterone. In our litigious society, we have to understand the position our doctors are in. If they let us take an active role in our treatment plan, we have to assure them that we won't try to blame them at some later date.

On the other hand, in your relationship with your doctor remember that you are the client. If your doctor isn't meeting your needs, you need to either work with him or her to correct this or switch doctors. Your health is your right, as is your freedom to change doctors. Don't let a sense of obligation, a fear of offending your doctor, or anything else prevent you from making a change if you feel you should. This is especially important when you have a chronic health concern that will keep you returning to your doctor regularly. Your relationship with your doctor is the foundation of your health and well-being. The wrong doctor may make it difficult—if not impossible—to return to wellness and optimal health.

Things to Remember

- Some of the negative side effects of nonbioidentical hormone products, such as Premarin and Prempro, appear to be related to the chemical alteration of these substances and haven't been proven to apply to bioidentical hormones.
- Progesterone should always be used with estrogen to counter estrogen's proliferative effects.
- HRT is not a one-size-fits-all treatment; different protocols are optimal for different women.
- Complete all of the tests and evaluations suggested in this chapter to determine your risk factors before starting on HRT.
- If you decide to start HRT, you need to have easy access to, and confidence in, your doctor.

Conclusion

In addition to useful information and helpful direction, what we really want you to take away from this book is a message of hope—hope that the aging process need not inevitably involve pain or illness and hope that you can feel better and even completely recover from any perimenopausal or menopausal discomfort you may be experiencing. If this book has helped you embrace the idea that you *can* successfully manage your own health and that you're not at the mercy of your doctor or the health care system, then you've already accomplished the most important step. Hope is a powerful state, lending strength and focus, both of which you'll need to draw on as you go forward.

To take full responsibility for your health, you may need to be more assertive than you usually are, requiring a departure from the nice, easy-to-manage, suffer-in-silence type of woman you might have been in your doctor's office before. If that description fits you, please read on. Asking for things specifically and firmly doesn't have to mean resorting to disrespectful, abrasive, or rude behavior. In fact, you can be perfectly polite, perfectly pleasant, and perfectly clear all at the same time.

An approach you may find useful is the simple "broken record" technique. All you have to do is repeat yourself over and over until you're taken seriously. Describe your feelings, using "I" statements, showing your doctor that you take responsibility for yourself (for example, "I would like my hormone levels tested"). Be firm and sure of yourself, and *don't* get emotional. Try to focus on positive goals, such as how exciting it will be to finally get quantifiable test results so you can balance your hormones, instead of focusing on your resentment of a doctor who's making the process harder than it needs to be. For example, if your doctor says your thyroid is fine even though you've lost a huge amount of hair and are inexorably gaining weight while eating very little, simply keep repeating (calmly and with a smile on your face) that you appreciate the input, but you really would like your thyroid hormone levels tested nonetheless.

It's human nature for all of us, including doctors, to take the easiest path when we're presented with a choice. If your doctor knows it will be necessary to explain to your insurance company why lab tests have been requested, the easiest path would be to not request them. But when you become a bigger obstacle than that call to the insurance company, you'll get the tests you need.

Hopefully this book has helped you understand your personal situation—your symptoms, your health history, and your risk factors—and in the process has given you a good idea of what your hormonal status is and what your options are. The next step in the process of reclaiming (or ensuring the continuation of) your good health is to obtain the quantified, incontrovertible evidence of your hormone levels that lab tests will provide. You can't make sense of what's going on in your body until you have that information in hand. Once you have this information, you can make educated decisions about what type of treatment is best for you.

Our sincere wish is that after working through this book you'll go forward armed with the information you need to regain or maintain your good health. Through methodical and wise application of everything you've learned here, combined with the cooperation of a good doctor, you can experience the same renewed vitality, energy, and joy that many women have been fortunate to rediscover. We wish you the best of health!

—Kathy and Dale

APPENDIX A

Symptoms at a Glance

In the Hormone Symptom Evaluation in chapter 3, you thought about and listed your symptoms, but in order to resolve them, it's important to understand what causes them. Many symptoms of hormonal imbalance may be caused by a combination of hormone deficiencies. The following explanations deal with the most common hormonal causes, but to get to the bottom of what may be causing your specific symptoms, consult with your doctor and undergo appropriate testing. See chapters 4 through 6 for details on testing hormone levels.

Use the table of contents below to help you find the symptoms that affect you. As you read through these explanations, focus on what applies to you. Use your journal to jot down anything you think will help you and your doctor better understand your health and hormonal status. Also, bear in mind that excess estrogen unbalanced by progesterone will always depress thyroid function, so if low thyroid is a potential cause of your symptom, you will also need to test estrogen and progesterone levels. For symptoms that can be common or transient, such as abdominal pain, fatigue, or sinus problems, the occasional incidence may not be indicative of hormonal balance; with this sort of symptom consider hormone involvement if the problem is *chronic*.

Contents

Abdominal pain 185
Abdominal weight gain 185
Acne 185
Alcohol cravings 185
Allergies 186
Anxiety or panic attacks 186
Asthma 187
Attention-deficit/hyperactivity disorder 187
Back or leg pain 187
Bladder problems 188
Bowel problems 188
Brain fog and memory problems 188
Breathing difficulty 189
Brittle, thin, ridged fingernails 189
Burning sensation in the mouth 189
Buzzing or ringing in the ears 189
Carpal tunnel syndrome 189
Cervical dysplasia 190
Chronic colds and illnesses 190
Chronic or severe infections 190
Cold hands and feet 191
Cold sweats 191
Constipation 191
Craving or eating strange substances 191
Dark circles under the eyes 191
Decreased sex drive 192
Deflated, sagging breasts 192
Depression 192
Diabetes 193
Difficulty concentrating 193
Dizziness 193
Dry eyes 193
Dry, thin skin 193
Early menopause 194

Easy bruising 194
Eczema or psoriasis 194
Elevated cholesterol 195
Endometriosis 195
Environmental sensitivity 196
Excess hair growth 196
Excessive fatigue 196
Eyes sensitive to sunlight 196
Feeling ill after chronic stress or a severe stressful event 197
Feeling of bugs crawling on the skin 197
Feeling socially isolated 197
Fibrocystic breast disease 197
Fibromyalgia 198
Flatulence 198
Fluid retention and bloating 198
Food cravings 198
Gallbladder problems 199
Gum and tooth problems 199
Hair loss 200
Headaches and migraines 200
Heart palpitations 200
Heart problems 201
Heartburn 201
Heavy menstrual bleeding 201
Heightened sensitivity to medications 201
Hemorrhoids 202
High blood pressure 202
Hot flashes or night sweats 202
Hypoglycemia 203
Infertility 203
Insomnia and sleep problems 203
Insulin resistance 204
Intolerance of cold or heat 204
Irritability and mood swings 205
Joint pain 205
Light or less frequent periods 206
Liver pain or swelling 206
Looking older than your age 206
Low basal body temperature 206
Low blood pressure 207
Memory problems 207
Menstrual irregularity 207
Mood swings 207
Muscle pain 207
Muscle weakness 207
Osteoporosis or osteopenia 207
Pain and numbness in the hands or wrists 208

Pain at the bottom of the back of the rib cage 208

Pain near the ovaries 208

Painful intercourse 208

Pale face and lips 209

Premenstrual syndrome (PMS) 209

Protruding eyes 209

Puffy skin 209

Red, flaky patches on the face 209

Restless legs syndrome 209

Scalloped or thick tongue 210

Shorter menstrual cycle, with heavy bleeding and/or clotting 210

Sinus problems 211

Sluggishness in the morning 211

Snoring 211

Sore, tender breasts 211

Stiffness and pain 212

Strange skin coloration 212

Strange thoughts and psychological problems 212

Swollen hands and feet 213

Symptoms of low thyroid made worse by thyroid hormone supplementation 213

Thickening of the neck or a lump under the Adam's apple 214

Thinning eyebrows 214

Tingling in the hands and feet 214

Tinnitus 214

Upset stomach 214

Urinary incontinence 214

Urinary tract infections 215

Uterine fibroids 215

Vaginal pain, itching, or dryness 215

Vision problems 215

Voice changes 216

Weak, slow, or soft pulse 216

Weight gain 216

Weight loss (unexplained) 217

Yeast infections 217

Yellowish skin and whites of the eyes 217

Abdominal pain: See Gallbladder problems.

Abdominal weight gain: Weight gain can obviously be a result of eating too much, but there are several other potential causes that should be explored if you haven't changed your eating habits and you're gaining weight only in your abdomen:

- Fluid retention.
- An enlarged uterus, which puts pressure on your digestive system and other organs.
- Ovarian cysts, which form around an egg follicle during ovulation. If the ovulation cycle isn't completed and the egg isn't released, the cyst may continue to grow, causing both pain and swelling.
- Fibroids, which are noncancerous growths of varying sizes that sometimes get very large. They're generally located in the uterus and begin with an abnormal cell that becomes stimulated by excess estrogen and grows more rapidly.
- Excess cortisol, which, in addition to causing fat buildup in the stomach, chest, and face, can also lead to other health problems, such as insulin resistance, heart disease, and type 2 diabetes.

Test levels of estrogen, progesterone, thyroid, and cortisol to determine if a hormone imbalance is the cause. You should also have a gynecological checkup (which may include a pelvic ultrasound) to check for fibroids or cysts.

Acne: Acne and pimples are common in perimenopausal women. It's well-known that hormones are a key factor in the development of acne, as evidenced by the increased incidence during puberty. These skin problems can be a result of increased production of androgens ("male hormones" such as testosterone) resulting from deficiency of progesterone (Vexiau and Chivot 2002) or estrogen. Lower levels of estrogen in perimenopause and menopause cause lower levels of SHBG (sex hormone binding globulin), which allows remaining levels of testosterone to be more available and active in the body, resulting in acne. Test levels of estrogen, testosterone, and progesterone to try to determine the root cause of this symptom.

Alcohol cravings: Adrenal fatigue and the resulting hypoglycemia appear to cause a predisposition for compulsive drinking. Cortisol, produced by the adrenal glands, is critical in maintaining blood sugar at adequate levels to meet the body's energy needs. When the adrenals are fatigued, cortisol levels drop and the body can't maintain normal blood sugar levels, which leads to hypoglycemia. Alcohol craving is caused by the body's desperate desire for additional energy that results from this adrenal malfunction. The alcohol gives a quick burst of blood sugar and energy but leads to further loss of adrenal function after the effects of the alcohol wear off, creating a vicious cycle. Long-term consumption of alcohol compounds the problem by causing further adrenal fatigue. Test cortisol levels to see if adrenal fatigue could be the root cause of this symptom.

Allergies: Many women experience allergies for the first time in their midforties. When the adrenal glands aren't functioning properly because of stress, diet, and/or a thyroid, estrogen, or progesterone deficiency, the body is much more susceptible to allergies, which involve an inflammatory response. Cortisol is the most powerful anti-inflammatory substance in the body, and when insufficient amounts are produced by your adrenal glands, allergic reactions become common. Estrogen may also be involved, as your sinus cavities are lined with mucous membranes, which require estrogen to maintain adequate moisture. When these membranes get dry, they don't function as well, making you more susceptible to allergies. Measure cortisol, as well as estrogen, progesterone, and thyroid hormone levels to see if low cortisol or other hormone deficiency or imbalance might be the root cause of this symptom. Also see Sinus problems.

Anxiety or panic attacks: The brain requires estrogen for proper functioning and progesterone for balance. In addition to its more beneficial neural functions, estrogen's stimulation of brain neurons can have the net effect of causing an anxious, excitable condition. Progesterone has an opposite, calming effect. When you don't have enough progesterone, unchallenged estrogen can cause agitation and anxiety. Low estrogen, on the other hand, affects mood and equanimity. Adrenals may also be a key factor in increased anxiety, especially with panic attacks. Adrenal fatigue is a progressive condition and starts with the adrenal glands overproducing adrenaline and cortisol in response to physical or emotional stress. If the stress continues, the adrenal glands start to wear out and don't produce enough adrenaline and cortisol. The body tries to correct the situation by forcing the adrenals into hyperactivity, causing spikes in adrenaline and cortisol production, which are experienced as anxiety and even panic. Lastly, low thyroid may also be to blame for nervous disorders such as anxiety. Brain cells have a higher concentration of thyroid receptors (T3) than any other tissues, so the brain requires sufficient levels of thyroid hormones to function properly (Smith et al. 2002). Test levels of estrogen, progesterone, thyroid, and cortisol to determine if an imbalance with one of these hormones may be the cause of this symptom.

Asthma: Estrogen and progesterone have been shown to have positive effects on pulmonary function and airway responsiveness. A drop in these hormones is associated with an increase in asthma (Haggerty et al. 2003). Thyroid hormone replacement has also proven to improve asthmatic conditions (Abdel Khalek et al. 1991). Test estrogen, progesterone, and thyroid to see whether reduced levels may be the root cause of this symptom.

Attention-deficit/hyperactivity disorder (ADHD): Thyroid dysfunction may be the cause of some cases of ADHD. Researchers at the University of Maryland School of Medicine found a correlation between symptoms of hyperactivity and impulsivity and resistance to thyroid hormones, characterized by elevated levels of serum T3 and T4, as well as normal or high concentrations of serum thyroid stimulating hormone (TSH) (ScienceDaily 1997).

Back or leg pain: The incidence of back pain and sciatica (pain along the large sciatic nerve, running from the lower back down the back of each leg) increases after age forty-five. Sciatica is usually caused by pressure on the sciatic nerve, which in turn may be caused by a disk problem, such as a ruptured, slipped, or herniated disk or a pinched nerve. One or more of the following sensations may occur as a result of sciatica: pain in the rear or leg that's worse when sitting; burning or tingling down the leg; weakness, numbness, or difficulty moving the leg or foot; a constant pain on one side of the rear; or a shooting pain that makes it difficult to stand up. Back pain generally starts when hormone levels drop, and clinical studies have shown that estrogen replacement therapy significantly reduces nighttime pain but has less effect on daytime pain (Kyllonen et al. 1999). Studies have also shown that progesterone plays a role in repairing nerves and renewing their protective sheaths, resulting in regeneration of nerve fibers (Koenig, Gong, and Pelissier 2000). Estrogen is necessary to create progesterone receptors, so if it's low, estrogen must be supplemented in order for the body to utilize progesterone effectively. Anecdotal reports suggest that replacement of progesterone and estrogen resolves back pain and sciatica completely.

Thyroid hormones are also critical to nerve health, so levels should be checked along with estrogen and progesterone to see if imbalances of any of these could be causing your pain (Schenker et al. 2003; Wang and Yang 2002). Replacing estrogen, progesterone, or thyroid hormones if low may resolve this problem.

Bladder problems: Estrogen is critical for optimal functioning of the bladder and urethra. Declining estrogen levels cause the lower urinary tract to thin, atrophy, and lose elasticity, diminishing the ability of the walls of the urethra and bladder to manage the flow of urine. The end result is urine leakage when you sneeze, laugh, or cough. Other possible results are a feeling of urgency, the need to frequently get up at night to urinate, and the feeling that you can't completely empty your bladder. Low estrogen may also result in frequent bladder and urinary tract infections (Hextall and Cardozo 2001). Estrogen receptors in the bladder are especially sensitive to any lowering of general estrogen levels in the body. Test estrogen to determine if low levels are causing chronic bladder problems. You may also want to test follicle stimulating hormone (FSH) to see if you're nearing (or in) menopause. Also see Urinary tract infections.

Bowel problems: Bowel problems can be caused by many different things. Irritable bowel syndrome, a disorder that interferes with the normal functioning of the large intestine, is characterized by a group of symptoms that includes cramps and abdominal pain, bloating, constipation, and diarrhea. Stress, diet, and allergies can be causes of this condition, but chronic bowel problems may also be caused by imbalances or deficiencies of cortisol, thyroid hormones, estrogen, and/or progesterone. Test levels of all of these hormones if you're experiencing chronic bowel problems. Also see Constipation.

Brain fog and memory problems: Cognitive dysfunction is a complex problem and may be caused by either a deficiency or an imbalance of estrogen, progesterone, or thyroid or adrenal hormones. Estrogen is critical to optimal brain function in many ways (Sherwin 2003): It increases blood flow and the supply of oxygen and glucose to the neurons (glucose is the major fuel source of the brain); keeps the blood-brain barrier working properly; protects neurons and stimulates new neuron growth; increases neurotransmitter levels; and decreases the generation of the substance thought to cause Alzheimer's (Sherwin 1999a). On the other hand, too much estrogen increases brain cell excitability, so when estrogen is insufficiently balanced by progesterone, your ability to focus can suffer. Thyroid function is also critical in concentration and memory. The slowed metabolism caused by low thyroid impacts the entire body, including the brain, where it can lead to memory loss and inability to process data. And finally, if the adrenals are producing too much or too little cortisol, you'll also experience impaired memory and cognition. Test levels of estrogen, progesterone, thyroid, and cortisol to determine if a hormone deficiency or imbalance may be the cause of this symptom.

Breathing difficulty: The sensation of not being able to breath in enough air, known as *dyspnea* or "air hunger," can be caused by low thyroid function. Hypothyroidism may cause weakness of the respiratory muscles, including the diaphragm (F. J. Martinez, Bermudez-Gomez, and Celli 1989; Laroche et al. 1988), or suboptimal heart and lung function (Hellermann and Kahaly 1996). Test thyroid hormone levels to see if a deficiency is the root cause of this symptom. Hyperthyroidism also affects breathing, making it more shallow and rapid (Pino-García et al. 1998).

Brittle, thin, ridged fingernails: Thyroid malfunction may produce brittle nails, splitting of the nail bed from the nail plate, or raised ridges along the nail. This symptom is very definitive for low thyroid even if lab results show "low normal" levels. Thyroid hormone supplementation should cause nails to start growing normally again (Pazos-Moura et al. 1998). Test thyroid hormone levels to see if a deficiency is the root cause of this symptom.

Burning sensation in the mouth: Burning mouth syndrome, a chronic burning sensation of the oral mucous membranes and especially of the tongue, occurs in women seven times more often than men, generally in the perimenopause and menopause age range. Many women afflicted with burning mouth syndrome also experience alterations in the sensation of taste, including sensing bitter or metallic tastes (or both) or changes in the intensity of taste perception. All of these symptoms respond favorably to estrogen and progesterone treatment, so they appear to be hormone related (Trombelli et al. 1992; Perno 2001). Test estrogen and progesterone levels. Balancing or supplementing estrogen and progesterone may resolve this problem.

Buzzing or ringing in the ears: See Tinnitus.

Carpal tunnel syndrome: This syndrome, which causes numbness, pain, and/or tingling in the wrists or hands, is common in people with low thyroid.

Mucopolysaccharides, a substance that accumulates abnormally in hypothyroidism, cause retention of fluid in connective tissues. This exacerbates the swelling and worsens the compression of the median nerve as it passes under the connective tissues overlying the wrist (Perez-Ruiz et al. 1995; Cakir et al. 2003). Muscle cramps in the hands are also common. Test thyroid hormone levels to see if a deficiency is the root cause of this symptom.

Cervical dysplasia: Cervical dysplasia is abnormal cell growth in the cervix and can lead to cancer. The most common catalyst of this condition is a viral infection caused by the human papillomavirus (HPV), a sexually transmitted disease. HPV is widespread and generally not tested for, as it doesn't cause problems for most of the women who have it. Another cause is unchallenged estrogen and deficient progesterone, which creates an environment that can facilitate cervical overgrowth and result in cervical dysplasia or even cancer. Low levels of estrogen or thyroid hormones may also be a factor, as both are critical to optimal immune function (Brabin 2002). Test estrogen, progesterone, and thyroid hormone levels, and also test for HPV, to try to determine the root cause of this condition.

Chronic colds and illnesses: Estrogen has been proven to be a powerful booster of immune function (Carlsten 2005); it also protects the body from potential aberrations of the immune system, which may lead to autoimmune or other diseases. Any time your hormonal balance is off-kilter, you're more susceptible to infections. Your thyroid gland also plays a crucial role in maintaining your body's immune system. It regulates the metabolic rate within each cell and directly influences over one hundred cellular enzymes. Low thyroid causes susceptibility to viral and bacterial infections, especially those of the respiratory system and urinary tract. Impaired adrenal function is another possible cause of repeated colds, coughs, or urinary tract infections and the tendency to catch whatever illness is going around, as well as slow wound healing (Kovacs 2005). Test levels of estrogen, progesterone, thyroid, and cortisol to determine if a hormone deficiency or imbalance may be the cause of this symptom.

Chronic or severe infections: Having chronic or severe infections is one of the most common causes of adrenal fatigue. How frequently you get infections, how severe they are, and how long they last are good indicators of adrenal involvement. Continuous infections are not only an indicator of adrenal fatigue, they also worsen any existing adrenal deficiency. A single serious infection, such as pneumonia, sinusitis, bronchitis, or mononucleosis, can trigger adrenal exhaustion. This is a potentially serious condition, because once the adrenals are exhausted, subsequent serious infections may be life threatening. Measure cortisol levels to see if they're low. Since estrogen and thyroid hormones are also important in optimal immune system function, measure levels of these hormones, as well, to determine whether a deficiency of either is involved in this symptom.

Cold hands and feet: Reduced circulation due to low thyroid function can cause chronically cold extremities. Because the thyroid regulates body temperature, suboptimal thyroid function generally causes intolerance to heat or cold. Test thyroid hormone levels to see if a deficiency is the root cause of this symptom. Also see Intolerance of cold or heat.

Cold sweats: See Hot flashes or night sweats.

Constipation: One of the primary causes of constipation is sluggish metabolism due to low thyroid, which slows the entire body down, including the digestive process. Low thyroid can also cause hemorrhoids. Low estrogen when you still have high levels of progesterone may also cause constipation (Pustorino et al. 2004; Deen, Seneviratne, and de Silva 1999). Test your estrogen and progesterone levels to determine if you have excessive unbalanced progesterone; also test thyroid function. Balancing estrogen and progesterone or replacing thyroid if low should resolve this problem.

Craving or eating strange substances: Also known as *pica*, craving or eating unusual substances such as ice, ashes, chalk, or starch can be a sign of low iron, which can cause anemia (Kushner and Shanta Retelny 2005). Perimenopausal women who have very heavy bleeding for several months should be on the lookout for signs of anemia and be tested regularly while bleeding continues. Test your estrogen and progesterone levels to see if you have an excess estrogen condition. Balancing estrogen and progesterone should resolve this problem.

Dark circles under the eyes: The most common cause of dark bluish circles under the eyes is nasal congestion, which can be caused by allergies triggered by adrenal fatigue (Marks 1977). The veins from the eyes drain into the veins of the nose. If the nose is blocked up, the veins around the eyes become larger and darker. This symptom may also be caused by chronic sinus infections or recurrent colds, which are also indicators of adrenal insufficiency. Test cortisol levels to determine if adrenal fatigue is causing this symptom.

Decreased sex drive: Declining estrogen levels can lead to a decrease in blood supply, which reduces functioning of nerves in the genital area (Ting, Blacklock, and Smith 2004). This causes a lack of clitoral sensitivity, as well as general numbing of the entire genital area, resulting in unsatisfying intercourse. All of your sexual organs require estrogen for a fulfilling sexual experience (Sherwin 1985). Progesterone is also critical for optimal sexual function, so progesterone deficiency could be at the root of a drop in sex drive. Thyroid has been found to be critical to libido and sexual performance, too (Carani et al. 2005). Finally, testosterone is also critical to proper functioning of the female genital system, including the nipples, the labia majora, and particularly the size and sensitivity of the clitoris. Test estrogen, progesterone, testosterone, and thyroid hormone levels. Replacement of these hormones, if low, should reverse this symptom.

Deflated, sagging breasts: Also called *breast ptosis*, this condition is caused by decreasing estrogen levels. Small breasts are a sign of lifelong low estrogen levels, but sagging, drooping breasts are a sign of excessive loss of estrogen later in life. Without adequate estrogen, the connective tissue of the breast becomes dehydrated and inelastic. The breast tissue, which was prepared to make milk, shrinks and loses shape, and its glandular tissue is reduced. Test estrogen levels to determine whether estrogen supplementation could be a solution.

Depression: There are many different kinds of depression, and this condition may be due to biological, psychological, inherited, or environmental factors, or a combination of them. That hormones are also involved in depression is indicated by several facts: Women have roughly twice the rate of depression as men, with approximately one in five women becoming clinically depressed during her lifetime (Regier et al. 1993). Also, many women being treated for depression are between the ages of twenty-five and fifty, the same age range in which women experience symptoms of hormone imbalance. Estrogen appears to play a major role in the formation of neurotransmitters in the brain, such as serotonin, which decreases depression, irritability, and anxiety. Decreasing estrogen levels may cause depression (Young et al. 2000; Sherwin 1994), and imbalances between estrogen and progesterone or low thyroid or adrenal function may also be involved (Piccirillo et al. 1994). Test estrogen, progesterone, thyroid, and cortisol to see if any hormone deficiencies or imbalances are contributing to this symptom. Also see Irritability and mood swings.

Diabetes: Characterized by elevated blood glucose (blood sugar), diabetes is the most common endocrine disorder. It is divided into two major subgroups. Type 1 diabetes is caused by insulin deficiency due to a malfunction of the cells in the pancreas that produce insulin. In type 2 diabetes the pancreas makes plenty of insulin, but the body's cells are resistant to its action, resulting in high blood sugar. Excess cortisol has been determined to be a primary cause of insulin resistance, which is a precursor to diabetes, so have your levels of cortisol tested to determine if high cortisol could be causing this disorder. Also see Insulin resistance.

Difficulty concentrating: See Brain fog and memory problems.

Dizziness: A very common hormonal cause of dizziness, or vertigo, is low estrogen. Low estrogen causes a decrease in blood flow and results in light-headedness and dizziness, which sometimes occur at the same time as other symptoms of low estrogen, such as hot flashes (Cali 1972). Test estrogen to determine if low levels are the cause of this symptom.

Dry eyes: Declining estrogen levels may result in less moisture in the tissue of the eyeballs. Estrogen receptors have been detected in the eyes, indicating that eye health is dependent on optimal estrogen levels. Clinical studies have shown that lack of estrogen causes pressure in the eyes, resulting in cataract formation, macular degeneration, and dry eyes. This can cause problems such as irritation and abrasion with contact lenses, which need sufficient moisture to buffer the lens from the eye (Lang et al. 2002; Jensen et al. 2000). Test estrogen to determine if low levels are causing your eyes to be unusually dry.

Dry, thin skin: Estrogen is critical for healthy and elastic skin. This largest organ of the body has extensive estrogen receptors and is dramatically affected by a drop in estrogen supply. Decreased estrogen also leads to reduced capillary blood flow, impeding delivery of oxygen and nutrients to the skin, as well as removal of wastes. Studies have shown that loss in elasticity and strength of skin due to declining levels of estrogen may be reversed with replacement of estrogen, which increases skin thickness and aids in collagen formation (Raine-Fenning, Brincat, and Muscat-Baron

2003; Vaillant and Callens 1996). Low thyroid is also a common cause of dry skin (Westphal 1997). Test estrogen and thyroid hormones to determine if low levels are causing this problem. You may also want to test follicle stimulating hormone (FSH) to see if you're nearing (or in) menopause.

Early menopause: Also called *premature ovarian failure,* early menopause can be caused by several different things. A common cause is autoimmune disease in which a woman develops antibodies to her own ovarian tissue, endometrium, or one or more of the hormones that regulate ovulation. These antibodies attack the reproductive system and compromise ovarian function. Genetic influences may also be involved. Having a family history of premature menopause (in your mother, grandmother, or sister) increases your chances of experiencing early menopause. Another genetic factor is an inherited defect on one of your X chromosomes that interferes with egg production. Viral infections are another possible cause. If a mother contracts a viral infection while pregnant with a baby girl, this can affect the baby's ovarian development, causing her to be born with a lower number of eggs than usual. This results in early depletion of eggs and premature menopause. On a related note, some people theorize that a small number of women may experience premature menopause if they had mumps and the infection spread to their ovaries. Lastly, long-term low thyroid function, causing inadequate functioning of all parts of the body, can profoundly affect ovarian function and cause the ovaries to shut down at an earlier age. Test estrogen, follicle stimulating hormone (FSH), and thyroid hormone levels to see if you are in early menopause and if significantly low thyroid function could be a factor.

Easy bruising: Easy bruising can be a sign of low thyroid (Tjan-Heijnen et al. 1994). Test thyroid hormone levels to see if a deficiency is the root cause of this symptom.

Eczema or psoriasis: Eczema, an acute or chronic inflammation of the skin, is characterized by redness, papules, pustules, scales, crusts, or scabs. Psoriasis, a chronic skin disease, manifests as red papules that join to form plaques with distinct borders. It can range from a minor cosmetic problem to a life-threatening condition. Skin disorders such as eczema and psoriasis are common in hypothyroidism (Hornstein 1984). Low cortisol levels can also be a complicating factor in both eczema and psoriasis. Test levels of thyroid hormones and cortisol to see if a deficiency of either may be the cause. Also test estrogen and progesterone, since unchecked estrogen can cause hypothyroidism.

Elevated cholesterol: Estrogen has many protective cardiovascular functions, including helping prevent elevated cholesterol. When present in sufficient amounts, estrogen lowers LDL ("bad" cholesterol) by increasing its breakdown and elimination via the liver; increasing production of HDL (the type of cholesterol that takes plaque away from artery walls to the liver for excretion); improving blood flow in the body; and decreasing the formation of blood clots. Clinical studies have shown that patients with high cholesterol can be successfully treated by supplementing with hormones to mimic youthful levels (Lobo 1990). Several studies have also shown positive effects of estrogen replacement therapy on cardiovascular risk (Eriksson et al. 1999). Low thyroid function can also lead to elevated levels of LDL and homocysteine (an amino acid linked to heart disease). Lowered metabolism due to low thyroid allows cholesterol to build up in the arteries and cause atherosclerosis (Pearce 2004; Duntas 2002). Test levels of estrogen and thyroid to determine if an imbalance with one of these hormones may be the cause of this symptom.

Endometriosis: This is a condition where tissue and cells from the inner lining of the uterus, or endometrium, grow outside the walls of the uterus in areas such as the bladder, intestines, abdomen, and ovaries. During menstrual flow, blood is released from these other growths, but has no outlet as in uterine bleeding. It causes inflammation and severe pain, particularly during intercourse or bowel movements. The number of women with endometriosis is growing dramatically. It is found in approximately 5 to 10 percent of reproductively viable women and 25 to 50 percent of infertile women (Brandt 2006). Standard treatment is prescription of birth control pills containing synthetic progestins, pain medication such as ibuprofen, or surgery to remove the growths, often along with the ovaries, uterus, and fallopian tubes. Endometriosis frequently causes infertility, but if you are able to get pregnant, it almost always disappears during pregnancy, when progesterone levels are extremely high. Many doctors use progesterone supplementation to treat it and temper the continual cell proliferation caused by estrogen. It may also be related to autoimmunity and thyroid disease, as women with endometriosis are more likely to suffer from various autoimmune diseases as well as hypothyroidism, chronic fatigue syndrome, fibromyalgia, lupus, multiple sclerosis, asthma, or allergies. Test levels of estrogen, progesterone, and thyroid hormones to determine the root cause.

Environmental sensitivity: Sensitivity to environmental factors, such as smog, chemicals, and scents, is generally caused by adrenal fatigue. If your adrenals aren't functioning well, you won't be able to tolerate these odors and they'll tax your body. This can actually be the catalyst for further adrenal fatigue. Low estrogen is another potential cause of chemical sensitivities and increased allergies. Measure estrogen and cortisol to see if either is low and may be causing this symptom. Also see Allergies.

Excess hair growth: As their hormone levels change, some women grow increased facial and body hair and find that the hair on their limbs becomes thicker and darker. Altered levels of androgens ("male hormones") are the most common cause of excessive hair growth, or hirsutism (Morrow 1977). Estrogen reduces the effects of androgens in women by increasing levels of SHBG (sex hormone binding globulin), which controls androgen levels to a degree. Thus, lack of estrogen effectively increases available blood androgens. Progesterone plays an important role, too, because it helps modulate other hormones and restore balance. Progesterone supplementation has been successful in reducing hair growth. If adequate estrogen isn't produced, supplementing with estrogen (as well as progesterone) should be considered. Test levels of estrogen, progesterone, and testosterone (an androgen) to try to determine the root cause of this symptom.

Excessive fatigue: There are many causes of excessive fatigue. The first is hypothyroidism, explained in detail in chapter 5. Another possible cause is fibromyalgia, a disease characterized by a profound degree of fatigue and generalized pain, with disturbances of mood and sleep. Recent research findings suggest that fibromyalgia is caused by inadequate regulation of cell function by thyroid hormones (Lowe 2000). Thyroid hormone deficiency and/or partial cellular resistance to thyroid hormones is thought to be genetic and/or environmental in origin. Adrenal dysfunction, covered in detail in chapter 6, may also cause chronic exhaustion (Di Giorgio et al. 2005; Jefferies 1994). Lastly, very low estrogen levels may result in significant fatigue. Test levels of estrogen, progesterone, thyroid, and cortisol to see if an imbalance with one of these hormones is the cause of this symptom. HRT may be necessary to correct this problem if levels are deficient.

Eyes sensitive to sunlight: When you're suffering from adrenal fatigue, your pupils can't stay effectively contracted, so the eyes become very sensitive to sunlight. This symptom is very accurate for detecting profound adrenal fatigue. Try the adrenal self-tests in chapter 6 to see whether adrenal function may be the cause, and if it seems to be, measure cortisol levels to accurately diagnose what's going on.

Feeling ill after chronic stress or a severe stressful event: The adrenals play an important role in helping you respond to stress, so when they're fatigued, you may have a hard time coping with stress or even actually feel ill or shaken in response to stress. The more frequently you're stressed or the greater the stressor is, such as a divorce or the death of someone close to you, the greater your chance of adrenal malfunction. All of the stressors you experience, whether due to personality, environmental conditions, illness or accidents, or life events, add up to deplete your adrenal function. Even when the individual stressors are quite unrelated, such as getting a bronchial infection, being promoted at work, and then getting married, stress is cumulative, so it can be hard to see the influence of stressful situations in draining your adrenal reserves. Measure cortisol levels to see if adrenal fatigue is causing this symptom.

Feeling of bugs crawling on the skin: The sensation of ants or bugs crawling on the body is called *formication*, from the Latin word *formicatio*, meaning "to creep like an ant." This symptom sometimes occurs along with feelings of vibration and appears to be related to increased sensitivity of nerve endings as estrogen levels decline. Test estrogen to determine if low levels are causing this. You may also want to test follicle stimulating hormone (FSH) to see if you're getting low on eggs and nearing menopause.

Feeling socially isolated: See Strange thoughts and psychological problems.

Fibrocystic breast disease: Because breasts have so many estrogen and progesterone receptors, some amount of tenderness and swelling is normal at the times in your menstrual cycle when hormone production peaks. But if you're no longer ovulating regularly, the discomfort gets worse because of fibrocystic activity, which causes breast tissue to become lumpy due to thickened connective tissue or small cysts. This may continue the entire month, growing increasingly painful during anovulatory cycles. This condition, known as *fibrocystic breast disease*, makes many women worry about breast cancer. The good news is that breast cancer almost never causes pain in the breasts, so if your breasts are tender, cancer probably isn't involved. But the condition is still of concern because chronic excess estrogen, together with deficient progesterone, is a breast cancer risk factor. Progesterone has been demonstrated to dramatically decrease cell multiplication, and studies have shown progesterone to be a promising treatment for breast cancer (Formby and Wiley 1998). Low thyroid (and/or deficient iodine) has been found to cause fibrocystic breast disease (L. Martinez et al. 1995). Clinical data has also shown a close link between low thyroid, fibrocystic breast disease, and an increased risk of breast cancer (Vorherr 1986). Test your estrogen and progesterone levels to determine if you have excess estrogen, and also test thyroid function. Balancing estrogen and progesterone, or replacing thyroid hormones or iodine if low, may resolve fibrocystic breast disease. Also see Sore, tender breasts.

Fibromyalgia: This disease is characterized by a profound degree of fatigue, disturbances of mood and sleep, and generalized pain. Recent, significant research findings suggest that fibromyalgia is caused by inadequate thyroid hormone regulation of cell function. This basic thyroid hormone deficiency or partial cellular resistance to thyroid hormones is thought to be genetic and/or environmental in origin. When cellular thyroid resistance is involved, thyroid tests will generally show normal thyroid levels, so the only way to determine if this is a potential solution for you is to cautiously try thyroid supplementation and see if your condition responds. You should measure thyroid hormone levels, as well, to see if they're low. Also see Excessive fatigue.

Flatulence: See Gallbladder problems.

Fluid retention and bloating: Progesterone, which functions as a natural diuretic, eliminates excess fluid and tempers the bloating effect of estrogen. When progesterone levels are low due to anovulatory cycles, chronic unbalanced estrogen causes fluid retention and results in swollen hands and feet. This condition also causes the body to retain salt, which further exacerbates fluid retention. Test estrogen and progesterone levels to see whether an imbalance is causing this symptom. If it is, supplementing progesterone in the last two weeks of the cycle should resolve this condition quickly. Hypothyroidism can also cause a form of puffiness and swelling, called *myxedema*, so you should also test thyroid hormone levels.

Food cravings: Food cravings are often physiological and not just due to lack of willpower. When excess estrogen is unchecked in your system because you don't have enough progesterone to balance it, your body attempts to balance the estrogen by producing more progesterone. One of the things it requires to manufacture progesterone is magnesium, so you may crave foods high in this mineral, such as chocolate. Another possible cause is low thyroid function, which has many causes, including unchecked estrogen. Hypothyroidism decreases your body's ability to use fats, proteins, and carbohydrates. When your body doesn't get what it needs, it responds with increased appetite and food cravings. If your adrenals are fatigued, you'll crave simple sugars and carbohydrates, which can raise blood sugar levels temporarily. Although this makes you feel better for a short time, it sets off a chain reaction wherein high blood sugar triggers the release of insulin, resulting in your blood sugar level crashing. Then you crave more sugar and carbohydrates to bring it back up again. Test levels of estrogen, progesterone, thyroid hormones, and cortisol to determine if a hormone imbalance may be the cause of this symptom.

Gallbladder problems: Unchallenged estrogen may exacerbate gallbladder problems, the most common digestive disease in the United States, currently affecting over twenty million people (Everhart et al. 1999). Bloating, gas, nausea, and pain that gets worse after eating, particularly fried foods, are all signs of gallbladder disease, which doctors refer to as the "four Fs"—female, fertile, forty, and flatulent. Bile is made in the liver and then stored in the gallbladder, a small pear-shaped organ located on the underside of the liver, until needed for the digestion of fat. When gallstones form, the bile duct can actually get blocked, causing an emergency situation requiring surgery. Both estrogen and progesterone are involved in adequate flow of bile to keep the gallbladder functioning properly, as indicated by research showing that there are both estrogen and progesterone receptors in the gallbladder (Singletary, Van Thiel, and Eagon 1986), making it very sensitive to hormone fluctuations. Test levels of estrogen and progesterone to determine if an imbalance is causing this problem.

Gum and tooth problems: Estrogen receptors in the gums and other tissues in the mouth indicate that estrogen plays a role in gum and tooth health. Gum recession and periodontal disease often occur as estrogen levels decline, and both of these conditions can also affect the teeth. Replacing estrogen along with appropriate levels of progesterone has been successful in reversing these conditions. Test estrogen to determine if low levels are causing gum and tooth problems. Addressing this problem may be more important than you realize, as subclinical dental infections can play a role in a wide variety of chronic health problems, including heart disease (Lopez-Marcos, Garcia-Valle, and Garcia-Iglesias 2005; Pelissier 1998).

Hair loss: High levels of testosterone in relation to estrogen may cause male-pattern baldness. Hypothyroidism can also cause hair loss, but in a different pattern, leading to thinning over the whole scalp, as well as loss of body hair. Declining estrogen can also cause hair loss (Fistarol 2002; Raine-Fenning, Brincat, and Muscat-Baron 2003). Test estrogen, progesterone, testosterone, and thyroid hormone levels. Supplementing any deficiencies or correcting any imbalances among these hormones should resolve this problem.

Headaches and migraines: Three out of four people suffering migraines are women, particularly those between the ages of thirty-five and forty-five. There's evidence that low or fluctuating estrogen levels can trigger migraines, particularly as women most commonly get them right before or right after their periods, when estrogen levels are lowest (Recober and Geweke 2005). As in all other conditions caused by an imbalance between estrogen and progesterone, if your progesterone is too low to balance your estrogen, the swelling caused by unchallenged estrogen can also be a catalyst. Interestingly, many women experience their first migraines when they begin taking birth control pills, a medication that alters hormonal balance. Nonmigraine headaches are also very prevalent in perimenopause and can be caused by arterial spasms due to insufficient levels of magnesium. One possible cause of insufficient magnesium is a chronic abundance of estrogen relative to progesterone. Low thyroid or low adrenal function can also cause headaches (Silberstein 1992a, 1992b). Interesting research from the 1920s found that low ovarian function caused the pituitary to become hyperactive, resulting in an actual increase in the size of the pituitary, which occupies a very limited bony space. This increase in size causes intracranial tension and pressure headaches (Harrower 1922). Supplementing estrogen may resolve this stimulatory effect on the pituitary gland and resolve this type of headache. To get to the root of this problem, test your levels of estrogen, progesterone, thyroid, cortisol, and magnesium (a red cell magnesium test that measures intracellular magnesium level is best).

Heart palpitations: Heart palpitations are the sensation of irregular, skipped, or rapid heartbeats. Although palpitations are very common and often harmless, they can be frightening, and sometimes they're a symptom of a serious problem. Heart palpitations may be caused by falling estrogen levels (Rosano, Leonardo, et al. 2000) or either low or high levels of thyroid hormones. Test levels of estrogen and thyroid to try to determine the root cause of this symptom.

Heart problems: Estrogen is important to the health of your heart in several ways. It helps protect the linings of the arteries from free radical damage, keeping them healthy and flexible so blood can flow freely. It also increases production of "good" cholesterol (HDL), which helps to remove "bad" cholesterol (LDL) from your system. This means less plaque formation and less clogging of the arteries as a result. The Postmenopausal Estrogen/Progestin Interventions (PEPI) Trial found that estrogen replacement therapy raised the level of HDL and lowered LDL (Abrams 1995). Although subsequent clinical studies have produced conflicting results, it's generally recognized that estrogen replacement is beneficial for your heart. Thyroid hormones are also involved in cardiovascular disease because of their important role in fat metabolism. Blood levels of triglycerides and cholesterol increase with hypothyroidism and decrease with hyperthyroidism. Test thyroid hormones and estrogen levels to see whether either is the root cause of this symptom. Also see Elevated cholesterol, Heart palpitations, and High blood pressure.

Heartburn: Heartburn is very common in perimenopausal women. Sometimes heartburn is a side effect of gallbladder problems, which may be exacerbated by unchallenged estrogen. Gastroesophageal reflux, which causes pain and heartburn, has also been shown to be affected by estrogen imbalance (Nilsson et al. 2003). Test levels of estrogen and progesterone to try to determine the root cause of this symptom. Also see Gallbladder problems.

Heavy menstrual bleeding: See Shorter menstrual cycle, with heavy bleeding and/or clotting.

Heightened sensitivity to medications: When your thyroid isn't functioning optimally, all of your metabolic activities slow down, including your liver function. The liver plays a central role in the detoxification process, and your body ultimately views most drugs as toxins. To clear them from your body, they're taken up by your liver, degraded, and excreted, so if your liver isn't working well, you become oversensitive to all medications. Test thyroid hormone levels to see if hypothyroidism is causing this symptom.

Hemorrhoids: See Constipation.

High blood pressure: There are many causes of high blood pressure, or hypertension, and hormone imbalance is one of them. Unchallenged estrogen due to low progesterone causes retention of fluid, which can contribute to high blood pressure. Low levels of estrogen may also cause high blood pressure, as estrogen is instrumental in heart function: It lowers LDL (as does thyroid hormone) by increasing its breakdown and elimination through the liver; increasing production of HDL (the type of cholesterol that takes plaque away from artery walls to the liver for excretion); improving blood flow; and decreasing the formation of blood clots (Aldrighi et al. 2004). Hypothyroidism is also a major cause of high blood pressure since it can slow the heart rate to less than sixty beats per minute, reduce the heart's pumping capacity, and increase the stiffness of blood vessel walls. All of these may lead to high blood pressure (Rylance et al. 1985). Thyroid hormone levels should always be checked if you have elevated blood pressure. The adrenal glands also produce several hormones, including aldosterone and cortisol, which help regulate blood pressure. Therefore, disorders of the adrenal glands can affect your blood pressure, so levels of cortisol and aldosterone should be measured. Also check estrogen levels to see if an imbalance or deficiency could be causing this symptom.

Hot flashes or night sweats: Hot flashes cause intense sweating for one to five minutes. Some women have them hourly, and some very infrequently. They generally continue for about two years, but some women may have them for ten or even twenty years after menopause. Thinner women are more likely to have them because they don't have enough fat in which to make estrone after ovarian production of estradiol drops. About 25 percent of women experiencing hormonal imbalances suffer debilitating hot flashes, affecting work, home life, and sleep (Staropoli et al. 1998). Because sleep deprivation is a common consequence of hot flashes, insomnia and depression become part of the picture. Many women also report having cold flashes, where they suddenly feel clammy or chilled but still sweat, and even shiver and shake as though they have a fever. Some women report certain sensations just before a hot flash: the feeling of an electric shock under the skin or in the head or the sensation of a rubber band snapping between the skin and muscle. All of these symptoms signal your body's reaction to an increasing imbalance in hormone levels and a drop in estrogen levels (Sherwin and Gelfand 1984; Leonetti, Longo, and Anasti 1999;

Charkoudian 2003). Test your estrogen levels to see if they're extremely low; if they are, HRT should resolve the problem.

Hypoglycemia: Also called low blood sugar, hypoglycemia occurs when your blood sugar level drops too low to provide enough energy for your body's activities. One common cause of hypoglycemia is insulin resistance, a condition in which refined carbohydrates and sugars are converted to fat instead of being burned as fuel. Eating these foods triggers a chain reaction in which blood sugar levels spike and then crash, making your body ravenous for all the wrong foods once again. Insulin resistance is sometimes a result of elevated cortisol levels, which in turn may be a result of declining estrogen. Since high cortisol levels also make your body less sensitive to estrogen and thyroid hormones, the remaining levels you have can't be used as effectively. Test cortisol levels to see if impaired adrenal function might be causing this symptom. Also check levels of thyroid, estrogen, and progesterone to see if deficiencies or imbalances of any of these hormones may be a factor in your adrenal dysfunction.

Infertility: Fertility levels definitely decrease with age, so delaying having children can be a factor in infertility. In recent years, doctors have found that women are having anovulatory cycles at earlier and earlier ages. Since women continue to menstruate when they don't ovulate, there's no obvious sign of hormonal imbalance. But without ovulation to produce an egg, you can't get pregnant. Researchers are studying environmental causes linked to chemicals that can interrupt the function of the hypothalamus gland, which is responsible for regulating sex hormones and, thus, triggering ovulation. Low levels of progesterone, or luteal phase defect, is another possible cause of infertility (Lessey 2003; Tulpppala et al. 1991). Low thyroid could also be involved, as it results in infertility (in either the man or woman) and increased incidence of miscarriages (Jefferies 1996). Test your estrogen and progesterone levels to determine if you have an imbalance between estrogen and progesterone or a progesterone deficiency. Also test your thyroid function. The problem may be resolved by balancing estrogen and progesterone or replacing thyroid if it's low.

Insomnia and sleep problems: Sleep problems are a natural side effect of estrogen or progesterone deficiencies. A common problem caused by estrogen deficiency is hot flashes, which not only cause physical discomfort, but also interfere with your deep sleep phase. Deep sleep is crucial to overall good health, especially muscle and nerve repair. Sufficient progesterone is also critical to sleep, as unchallenged estrogen causes excitability and progesterone tempers it and promotes sleep. If progesterone or estrogen is deficient or imbalanced, your ability to fall asleep and stay asleep can be dramatically affected (Krystal 2004). Thyroid or cortisol excess or deficiency may also result in insomnia. Test estrogen, progesterone, thyroid, and cortisol to try to determine the root cause of this symptom.

Insulin resistance: This condition, which is a precursor of type 2 diabetes, results in a pattern of high levels of glucose and insulin in the bloodstream, which causes glucose to be stored as fat instead of being used for energy by muscle cells. Here's how it works: Glucose, or blood sugar, goes up after eating; insulin is then produced in order to utilize the glucose to be used by muscle or stored as fat. The insulin level is then supposed to drop quickly to its normal low level. As we get older and have less estrogen and more body fat, our insulin receptors become less functional and the body can't handle glucose as effectively. When the brain detects continued high glucose levels, it signals the pancreas to release even more insulin to lower the blood sugar level. As a result, blood sugar levels plummet, leading to a condition called *reactive hypoglycemia*, which makes the body ravenous for all the wrong foods to try to bring the blood sugar level up quickly.

Insulin resistance, which can be triggered or exacerbated by high cortisol levels, causes significant weight gain as well as compromised immune function and increased risk of heart disease. Estrogen deficiency is a critical component of the situation, as it is important in optimizing insulin response in the cells. Test levels of cortisol and estrogen (as well as progesterone for proper balancing). If estrogen is low, you might consider estrogen replacement therapy, but the most effective strategy for reversing this condition is a diet free of sugar and refined carbohydrates. Instead, choose whole grains and other complex carbohydrates and foods with a high protein content. Also see Diabetes.

Intolerance of cold or heat: Low thyroid function affects the body's ability to regulate body temperature, which makes a cold or hot environment much more uncomfortable. It also leads to reduced circulation, which causes chronically cold hands and feet. In some cases, the skin may receive as little as 20 to 40 percent of its normal blood supply, interfering with the body's ability to warm the extremities.

Irritability and mood swings: Estrogen stimulates brain neurons and progesterone calms them (Sherwin 1999b). Both are necessary—in the proper balance—to regulate your mood, as well as for overall health. If excess estrogen goes unchecked by progesterone, mood swings occur (Gruber et al. 1999). To make things confusing, however, deficient estrogen may also be at the root of irritability, as it has been shown to be essential in all aspects of brain function (Sherwin 1996). The bottom line is that too much or too little of either estrogen or progesterone can cause irritability and mood swings. Estrogen is commonly used to treat symptoms of depression and mood disorders during perimenopause and PMS (Gregoire et al. 1996).

Thyroid hormones and cortisol are also critical to mood and emotional stability. Adequate cortisol is important in curbing anxiety, moodiness, and excessive emotions, especially in stressful situations. Hyperthyroidism and hypothyroidism may be accompanied by psychiatric disturbances that can mimic mental illness. Hyperthyroidism can cause marked anxiety and tension, emotional instability, impatience, irritability, overactivity, and exaggerated sensitivity to noise. It can also cause fluctuating depression characterized by sadness and problems with sleep and appetite, and those with severe hyperthyroidism may even mimic schizophrenia by losing touch with reality, becoming delirious, or hallucinating. Hypothyroidism can lead to slowing of mental function, loss of interest and initiative, poor memory, general intellectual deterioration, depression, and paranoia. It can ultimately cause dementia and permanent damage to the brain. Many people with severe cases of thyroid malfunction have been wrongly diagnosed and hospitalized for psychosis. Test levels of estrogen, progesterone, cortisol, and thyroid hormones to see if imbalances in any of these hormones may be involved. Also see Anxiety or panic attacks and Depression.

Joint pain: Pain and swelling of joints may be caused by chronic strain or trauma to the joint, or it may be caused by an inflammatory response coupled with inadequate levels of cortisol (Cutolo and Masi 2005). This condition is usually misdiagnosed as arthritis and treated with anti-inflammatory drugs, like ibuprofen. These drugs reduce symptoms but generally cause serious side effects, such as gastrointestinal bleeding, ulcers, and kidney problems; plus, they don't stop progression of the condition. Supplementation with low-dose cortisol has been shown to relieve pain and swelling. Low estrogen can also result in widespread aches and pains, and estrogen replacement can make a profound contribution to reducing pain. Estrogen also increases production of serotonin, which blunts our response to pain signals from the body (Rybaczyk et al. 2005). Low thyroid may also be to blame, as it can cause shooting pains, often in the hands and feet (Punzi et al. 2002). Test levels of estrogen, progesterone, thyroid, and cortisol to determine if a hormone deficiency or imbalance may be the cause of this symptom. Also see Stiffness and pain.

Light or less frequent periods: As estrogen diminishes (generally somewhere between age forty and fifty), the time between your periods may start to lengthen, or you may even skip periods altogether. Estrogen is responsible for the growth of endometrial tissue, which then sloughs off to create your menstrual period. When estrogen levels drop, you don't make enough estrogen to build up your uterine lining, so your flow is much lighter. Test estrogen levels to see if low levels are causing this. You may also want to test follicle stimulating hormone (FSH) to see if you're getting low on eggs and nearing menopause.

Liver pain or swelling: Low levels of thyroid hormones cause liver function to slow down, which can result in swelling and pain in the area of the liver (the right side of the abdomen just under the rib cage). But there are many other causes of liver pain and swelling; the most common is liver disease caused by alcoholism. If you have this symptom, do the liver test in chapter 6 and test thyroid hormone levels to see if a deficiency is the root cause of this symptom.

Looking older than your age: Estrogen is critical in the regeneration of new cells and the breaking down of old ones. When the ovaries stop making estrogen, cell regeneration is slowed drastically, a hallmark of aging. Accelerated aging may also be due to hormone imbalances. Unchallenged estrogen, deficient progesterone, adrenal fatigue, and low thyroid are all conditions that can cause premature aging. The first step is always to balance estrogen and progesterone. This restores the body's basic rhythm and allows you to see if the functioning of other hormones and glands, such as the thyroid and the adrenals, will normalize. Test levels of estrogen, progesterone, thyroid, and cortisol to determine if hormone imbalance may be the cause of this symptom.

Low basal body temperature: Lowered metabolism due to low thyroid function is one of the main reasons for a basal body temperature lower than 97.8°F. Two other reasons for low body temperature are liver disease and alcoholism. Test thyroid hormone levels to see if a thyroid deficiency is causing this symptom.

Low blood pressure: Low adrenal function is a common cause of low blood pressure, although it can also be caused by other conditions, such as infections and heart disease. Low blood pressure due to adrenal insufficiency can be diagnosed by testing your blood pressure while lying down and then again immediately on rising. If it drops when you move from a lying to a standing position, it's almost always an indication of low adrenal function. (See chapter 6 for more details on this self-test.) Low thyroid is also a common cause of low blood pressure, due to a lowered metabolic rate throughout the body. Test levels of thyroid and cortisol to determine if a deficiency in one of these hormones may be the cause of this symptom.

Memory problems: See Brain fog and memory problems.

Menstrual irregularity: See Light or less frequent periods and Shorter menstrual cycle, with heavy bleeding and/or clotting.

Mood swings: See Irritability and mood swings.

Muscle pain: See Stiffness and pain.

Muscle weakness: If cortisol is too high, large amounts of muscle protein are broken down to produce amino acids, which are then converted into glucose in the liver to be used as fuel. Weak muscles may indicate hypothyroidism, due to the lowered metabolic state it creates. Low estrogen can also cause muscle weakness and loss of muscle mass. Another possible cause is low testosterone levels, which lead to reduced muscle strength and volume. Test levels of estrogen, progesterone, testosterone, thyroid hormones, and cortisol to determine if a hormone deficiency or imbalance may be the cause of this symptom.

Osteoporosis or osteopenia: These are diseases of decreasing bone density and bone loss. In osteoporosis, bones are less dense and more fragile and thus at greater risk for fracture, even with just a small amount of trauma. *Osteopenia*, the term used for bones that have become somewhat less dense than normal, isn't as severe as osteoporosis. However, a person with osteopenia has a higher risk of developing osteoporosis. By age thirty-five, most women have started to lose bone, and losses usually become increasingly rapid after menopause. Risk factors include being thin and petite or Caucasian; smoking; eating a poor diet; chronically taking certain drugs, such as antacids, diuretics, or sleeping pills; or a genetic tendency (especially if your mother or another close relative has had problems with bone loss). Taking calcium isn't a solution for osteoporosis. Calcium is lost from the bones at such a rate that it can't be replaced by supplements. However, estrogen has been proven to slow the loss of bone (Gordan 1985; Carlsten 2005) and progesterone appears to be critical in ongoing building of new bone (I. U. Schmidt, Wakley, and Turner 2000). An analysis of twenty-two trials with data on a total of 8,800 women found a 27 percent reduction in risk of nonvertebral fractures in older women who received HRT (Grady and Cummings 2001). The few years right after onset of menopause may be the most important time to start using HRT, as bone loss is greatly accelerated during this period. Weight-bearing exercise has also been proven to slow bone mineral loss, or even improve density (Sinaki 1989). Test estrogen and progesterone to determine whether you're at risk for osteoporosis due to estrogen and progesterone deficiencies.

Pain and numbness in the hands or wrists: See Carpal tunnel syndrome and Joint pain.

Pain at the bottom of the back of the rib cage: The two adrenal glands sit on top of the kidneys, just underneath your last rib. They're about one inch high and one to two inches wide. When they aren't functioning correctly, they can actually become painful to the touch. Measure cortisol levels to see if adrenal fatigue is causing this symptom.

Pain near the ovaries: Midcycle pain in the region of your ovaries during ovulation (called *mittelschmerz*) is probably caused by the rupturing follicle releasing the egg for fertilization. When you fail to ovulate, a cyst may be formed that doesn't rupture, but the attempt to do so causes pain. Doctors often recommend surgery to remove this type of cyst. If it grows too large and resists other treatment, this may be necessary, but the first and least invasive solution to try is normalizing the menstrual cycle by using progesterone during the last two weeks of the cycle. Hypothyroidism also causes many menstrual irregularities and can be the catalyst for this symptom. Test levels of estrogen, progesterone, and thyroid hormones to try to determine the root cause of this symptom.

Painful intercourse: The vagina is highly estrogen dependent. When levels drop, the vagina's cells thin, leading to dryness, loss of elasticity, and reduced mucus production. This may ultimately result in up to 90 percent loss of thickness and elasticity and can lead to discomfort during intercourse (Hextall and Cardozo 2001; Ting, Blacklock, and Smith 2004). Test estrogen to determine if low levels are causing this. You may also want to test follicle stimulating hormone (FSH) to see if you're getting low on eggs and nearing menopause. Also see Vaginal pain, itching, or dryness.

Pale face and lips: Reduced circulation and vasodilation due to hypothyroidism may be the cause of this symptom. Test thyroid levels to see if this is the root cause. This symptom often occurs when low adrenal function accompanies low thyroid function.

Premenstrual syndrome (PMS): Almost one-third of all women experience some level of PMS. The most common symptoms are breast lumps and tenderness, headaches, cramps and pain, fatigue, bloating, fluid retention, weight gain, irritability, and mood swings. Deficiency of either estrogen or progesterone may be the cause. The adrenals can also play a part in PMS, as they are the backup source for estrogen and progesterone production when the ovaries start to sputter. So if the adrenals are already taxed at this time, they may not produce sufficient levels of estrogen and progesterone. Thyroid abnormalities have also been proven to cause PMS symptoms (P. J. Schmidt et al. 1993; Girdler, Pedersen, and Light 1995). Test levels of estrogen, progesterone, thyroid hormones, and cortisol to determine which of these hormones may be contributing to PMS symptoms.

Protruding eyes: Hyperthyroidism causes eyes to swell, a condition known as *exophthalmos*. Test thyroid hormone levels (and also consider testing thyroid antibody levels) to see if an overactive thyroid is the root cause of this symptom.

Puffy skin: Atypical puffiness, or a quilted appearance of the skin, called *myxedema*, can be caused by hypothyroidism (Ozawa 2005). The face and eyelids are often especially afflicted by this condition. Excess estrogen relative to progesterone can also cause fluid retention and bloating. Test estrogen, progesterone, and thyroid hormone levels to see if a deficiency or imbalance is the root cause of this symptom.

Red, flaky patches on the face: See Eczema or psoriasis.

Restless legs syndrome: Research has shown that restless legs syndrome is related to low thyroid hormone levels and is often one of the initial signs of hypothyroidism (Schlienger 1985). Other research has connected restless legs syndrome to low iron levels in the brain, and the syndrome may be caused by anemia stemming from extremely heavy menstrual bleeding, which is often due to excessive estrogen in relation to progesterone (Bon et al. 1996). Test estrogen and progesterone levels to determine whether you have an excess estrogen condition; also test thyroid function. Balancing estrogen and progesterone or replacing thyroid if low may resolve this problem.

Scalloped or thick tongue: This symptom can be caused by swelling, or edema, resulting from hypothyroidism (Reiss 1998). If you detect this symptom, have your thyroid hormone levels tested and supplement if your levels are low.

Shorter menstrual cycle, with heavy bleeding and/or clotting: Menstrual cycles are normally twenty-six to thirty-two days long, but the length may begin to change when you're still in your late twenties, with most women noticing a significant change by their midthirties to midforties. This change is caused by a shift in your hormone levels. When you don't ovulate, you don't make sufficient progesterone, so the lining of your uterus continues to grow, influenced by a steady stream of unchallenged estrogen. This causes you to have your period earlier than you normally would, often with very heavy bleeding, unusually long periods, or abnormal bleeding in the middle of your cycle (Hickey, Higham, and Fraser 2000; Lessey 2003). This heavy bleeding is often accompanied by painful cramps as large blood clots are expelled. Hypothyroidism is another cause of abnormal, excessive bleeding. The thyroid controls muscle contraction of the uterus. Without enough thyroid hormones, the muscles don't contract properly and the uterus doesn't effectively stop the blood vessels from bleeding (Wilansky and Greisman 1989).

For these symptoms, many doctors recommend a hysterectomy, endometrial ablation, or D&C, but balancing estrogen with progesterone or supplementing thyroid hormones may resolve the situation and should be considered first, before surgery (Irvine et al. 1998). Many doctors have found that intravaginal delivery of progesterone is most effective for this condition, as it specifically targets the uterus. As a precaution, you should also discuss with your doctor a diagnostic ultrasound to rule out uterine cancer, particularly if you've been having midcycle bleeding. This will test the thickness of your uterine lining and check for abnormalities. Test your estrogen and progesterone levels to see whether excess estrogen is involved. Anemia is a common side effect of heavier, clotted bleeding, so you also should have your iron levels checked. Check your thyroid hormone levels, too.

Sinus problems: Your sinus cavities are lined with mucous membranes, which require estrogen to maintain adequate moisture and function properly. When estrogen levels drop, your membranes get dry and aren't as effective in trapping and getting rid of bacteria and viruses, resulting in irritation and infections. The adrenal glands may also be involved in ongoing sinus problems, as they play an important role in mediating the histamine release and inflammatory reactions that produce allergy symptoms. Allergies, which are a major cause of sinus problems, may be caused by an overreaction of the immune system to relatively harmless allergens, such as dust or pollen. The immune system recognizes these as foreign substances and then mobilizes to destroy them, causing an inflammatory reaction. Adequate cortisol is key in reducing inflammation, so when you're not producing enough, you may get sinus problems and other symptoms of allergies. Test estrogen and cortisol to determine if a deficiency of either is causing this symptom. Also see Allergies.

Sluggishness in the morning: A pattern of having a hard time with getting going before ten in the morning may indicate adrenal insufficiency. The body's natural pattern is to produce the highest levels of cortisol first thing in the morning, so if your adrenals aren't making adequate levels of cortisol, you'll feel extremely tired when you first get up because your body is looking for that high initial peak. Thyroid hormones can also be involved in any unusual fatigue. Test levels of thyroid and cortisol to determine if a deficiency of either may be the cause of this symptom.

Snoring: There are many causes of snoring, including a narrow throat; excess weight and fatty tissue in the neck (which cause the throat to become smaller); nasal deformities, such as a deviated septum; narrowing of and decreased muscle tone in the throat due to aging; a history of smoking; enlarged adenoids or tonsils; a long soft palate or uvula; alcohol or medications such as sleeping pills or antihistamines, which increase relaxation of the throat and tongue muscles; allergies; asthma; or a cold or sinus infection. But there's also at least one hormonal factor: Snoring may also be caused by high blood pressure (Bixler et al. 2000), which may be due to low thyroid function or fluid retention as a result of unchallenged estrogen. Test your estrogen, progesterone, and thyroid hormone levels to determine whether you have an imbalance that may be involved in this problem. Also see High blood pressure.

Sore, tender breasts: Breasts have a large number of estrogen and progesterone receptors. When your estrogen or progesterone levels begin to rise (several weeks before your period, or shortly before your period, respectively), this can trigger soreness and swelling. During perimenopause, if your estrogen and progesterone levels are out of balance, the degree of tenderness and discomfort gets worse. If you're ovulating and producing enough progesterone to balance estrogen levels, the symptoms may go away until the week or two after your next period. If, on the other hand, your estrogen levels have decreased significantly while you're still ovulating, you may feel discomfort during the week before your period, when your progesterone levels are high. Measure your estrogen and progesterone levels to see whether an imbalance is involved in this symptom. Also see Fibrocystic breast disease.

Stiffness and pain: The low metabolic rate characteristic of hypothyroidism allows accumulation of metabolic waste products in the connective tissues of the joints, muscles, and ligaments, which can result in stiffness, aches, and pains. This is particularly noticeable in the neck and shoulders (Cakir et al. 2003). Low estrogen, or rapidly dropping levels of estrogen, can also result in muscle and joint pain. When estrogen levels are high, your brain responds more effectively to pain, releasing endorphins or enkephalins, chemicals that dampen the pain signals received by your brain. But when estrogen is low, pain isn't handled nearly as effectively. Test thyroid and estrogen levels to see if a deficiency of either is the root cause of this symptom. Also see Joint pain.

Strange skin coloration: Adrenal fatigue can cause discoloration of many different areas of the body: The pads of fat on the tips of the fingers or the palms often turn red. The inside of the lips, mouth, and vagina and the skin around the nipples may turn a bluish black color. The skin on scars, in folds of skin, around bony areas, and in the creases of joints may darken. And lighter-colored patches can develop in various spots, where the skin seems to have lost its usual coloration (Jabbour 2003). Measure cortisol levels to see if low adrenal function is causing this symptom.

Strange thoughts and psychological problems: Some of the psychological symptoms women have reported developing at perimenopause or menopause are anxious, agitated dreams; loss of confidence; obsessive, irrational patterns of thoughts and behavior; inability to multitask; social phobia, sense of loss of social skills, and withdrawal; grief and sadness with no cause; vocabulary and speech problems, such as difficulty with articulation and stammering; and "doom" thoughts, including feelings of dread and apprehension, sometimes involving thoughts of death or picturing one's own death. These wide-ranging effects may be due to deficiencies or imbalances of several hormones. Estrogen, which is essential to optimal brain function, has been shown to increase cerebral blood flow, enhance activity at neuronal synapses, act as an anti-inflammatory agent, and exert direct neuroprotective effects on the brain. Through these mechanisms, estrogen strongly influences cognition and mood, and the decline of estrogen levels at menopause can produce significant emotional and cognitive problems (Shepherd 2001). Estrogen and progesterone replacement therapy can improve brain function and resolve these symptoms. Thyroid hormones are also critical to normal mental function. Brain cells have more thyroid (T3) receptors than other tissues, so adequate levels of thyroid hormones are necessary for brain cells to function normally. Hyperthyroidism can also cause significant psychological problems, sometimes mimicking mental illness. Test levels of thyroid hormones, estrogen, and progesterone to try to determine the root cause of this symptom. Also see Anxiety or panic attacks, Depression, and Irritability and mood swings.

Swollen hands and feet: Swollen hands and feet, like a swollen abdomen, can be a sign of an imbalance between estrogen and progesterone. Excesses of either estrogen or progesterone can cause fluid retention (Stachenfeld and Taylor 2004). The key is to find out what your particular imbalance is—too much estrogen or too much progesterone. A helpful clue is noting when your symptoms get worse: two weeks before your period, right before your period, right after your period, or throughout your cycle. Hypothyroidism is another very common cause of fluid retention in the extremities, and often in the face and around the eyes, causing the skin to take on a puffy and almost quilted look. This kind of fluid retention generally dimples when you firmly press a finger to the area (Ozawa 2005). Test your estrogen, progesterone, and thyroid hormone levels. Balancing estrogen and progesterone or replacing thyroid hormones if low should resolve this problem.

Symptoms of low thyroid made worse by thyroid hormone supplementation: Long-term thyroid deficiency commonly results in eventual adrenal fatigue. Thyroid hormone therapy starts the body's metabolism back up, and as a result the liver begins to process hormones in the body more quickly. If adrenal fatigue is also a problem, once the body's existing stores of cortisol are used up the adrenals won't be able to produce sufficient additional quantities. This leads to symptoms of adrenal fatigue, with excessive fatigue being the primary symptom. Test cortisol levels to see if adrenal fatigue is the root cause of this symptom.

Thickening of the neck or a lump under the Adam's apple: This can be caused by a goiter, which is an enlargement of the thyroid gland caused by overactive or underactive thyroid function. It can cause choking, difficulty in swallowing, hoarseness, or a feeling of fullness in the neck. Test thyroid hormone levels to see if an overactive or underactive thyroid is the root cause of this symptom.

Thinning eyebrows: Thinning or loss of the hair at the ends of the eyebrows closest to the temples is a fairly definitive indicator of thyroid deficiency. Test thyroid hormone levels to see if a deficiency is the root cause of this symptom.

Tingling in the hands and feet: Imbalance between estrogen and progesterone or declining levels of estrogen can cause the feeling of pins and needles in the hands and feet, which is just one symptom of changes in nerves and muscles that cause blood vessels to constrict or dilate; hot flashes are also a result of this. Low thyroid function can also cause tingling in the extremities. Other, less likely reasons for this symptom include B_{12} deficiency, decreased flexibility of blood vessels, a depletion of calcium and/or potassium, or diabetes. Treatment depends on the cause, so test levels of B_{12}, calcium, and potassium, as well as levels of estrogen and progesterone to determine if you have an excess estrogen condition. Also test thyroid function and blood sugar levels (to see if diabetes is involved). Resolving any imbalance between estrogen and progesterone, replacing thyroid if low, and supplementing B_{12}, calcium, or potassium if deficient may solve this problem. Also see Carpal tunnel syndrome.

Tinnitus: Many women experience tinnitus, a condition characterized by ringing, buzzing, or whooshing sensations in the ears. It's associated with low thyroid and heart disease and is also a side effect of medications, including Prozac (fluoxetine) and aspirin (Elliott 2000). Test thyroid hormone levels to see if a deficiency is the cause of this symptom.

Upset stomach: Excess cortisol results in an increase in production of stomach acids, which can result in stomach upset and even ulcers. Test cortisol to see whether elevated levels are the root cause of a frequent or chronic upset stomach. Also see Bowel problems, Gallbladder problems, and Heartburn.

Urinary incontinence: See Bladder problems.

Urinary tract infections: When estrogen levels drop, the walls of the urinary tract thin out, weakening its mucous membranes and reducing their ability to resist bacteria. The bladder also loses elasticity and fails to empty completely, creating a breeding ground for bacteria. Estrogen loss also lessens immune function, which is important in blocking E coli from adhering to vaginal cells. Test estrogen levels and consider supplementing if your level is low. Also see Bladder problems.

Uterine fibroids: These noncancerous growths of varying sizes are generally located in the uterus. They begin with an abnormal cell that becomes stimulated by excess estrogen and grows more rapidly than surrounding cells. These growths can get very large (often the size of a grapefruit) and cause pelvic pressure, which can result in constipation, frequent urination, an enlarged abdomen, menstrual cramps, painful intercourse, and irregular, midcycle or very heavy bleeding. They are most common after age thirty and tend to shrink after menopause, when estrogen production drops off. Fibroids are very common; 20 to 40 percent of women over thirty-five develop them (American Family Physician 2000). Fibroids are the most common reason for hysterectomies. In fact, hysterectomies and removal of fibroids are two of the most commonly performed surgeries in the United States. Small fibroids generally respond well to progesterone therapy (particularly vaginal delivery of progesterone supplementation), which tempers the effects of estrogen, but surgery may be necessary for large fibroids. Surgical procedures have advanced greatly in recent years, so it should be possible to remove the fibroid via a laparoscopic procedure without removing the uterus (or other organs). Test levels of estrogen and progesterone to detect unchallenged estrogen.

Vaginal pain, itching, or dryness: Low estrogen leads to thinning of the tissue that lines the vagina and can cause vaginal pain, itching, or dryness. Test estrogen levels to determine if low levels are causing this. You may also want to test follicle stimulating hormone (FSH) to see if you're nearing (or in) menopause. Also see Painful intercourse.

Vision problems: Low levels of estrogen can cause eyesight problems (Yu et al. 2004) and have been linked to increases in macular degeneration, glaucoma, and cataracts. Test estrogen to determine if low levels are causing this. You may also want to test follicle stimulating hormone (FSH) to see if you're nearing menopause.

Voice changes: When estrogen levels decrease, many women's voices change in the following ways: decreased vocal intensity, increased vocal fatigue, decreased range, loss of high tones, and an overall loss of vocal quality. Clinical studies have proven that these changes are caused by loss of estrogen and that HRT can counteract them (Abitbol, Abitbol, and Abitbol 1999). Low levels of thyroid hormones sometimes cause hoarseness, making your voice sound weak, excessively breathy, scratchy, or husky. Test thyroid and estrogen levels to see if either is the root cause of this symptom.

Weak, slow, or soft pulse: Hypothyroidism is the primary cause of a weak, slow, or soft pulse. The low metabolic function caused by hypothyroidism slows all bodily functions, including pulse rate. This symptom can also be caused by low adrenal function. Check levels of thyroid hormones and cortisol and supplement either if your level is low.

Weight gain: Imbalance between estrogen and progesterone can be a factor in weight gain. Unchallenged estrogen causes weight gain at the hips and also decreases thyroid function, setting off a domino effect since a healthy thyroid is necessary for effective metabolism. Low thyroid may also be due to high levels of thyroid antibodies, which can seriously disrupt the thyroid's ability to regulate metabolism. The body's response to insufficient thyroid hormones is weight gain and accumulation of fat, particularly in the hips, thighs, abdomen, and buttocks. Cortisol, produced in response to physical or emotional stress, is another potential cause of weight gain. When your cortisol is too high, you store weight around the middle of your body, and until your cortisol levels normalize, this weight is impossible to lose (Andrew, Phillips, and Walker 1998; Bjorntorp and Rosmond 2000). There's another piece to the weight gain puzzle: Adrenal fatigue causes you to reach for foods that quickly raise your blood sugar and give you a burst of energy. Foods loaded with white flour and sugar are the most common culprits. Unfortunately, eating these foods can trigger a chain reaction, causing your blood sugar to spike and then crash, making you ravenous for all the wrong foods once again. This vicious cycle, called *insulin resistance*, can be dangerous to your health and lead to weight gain, compromised immune function, and increased risk of heart disease and type 2 diabetes. Also see Abdominal weight gain.

Weight loss (unexplained): One of the more common causes of unexplained weight loss is hyperthyroidism, which causes your metabolism to speed up, converting more of what you eat into energy. Test thyroid hormone levels to see if hyperthyroidism is involved.

Yeast infections: Yeast infections are caused by *Candida albicans*, a fungus that may grow in the vagina, mouth, or intestines. One of the factors encouraging the growth of this fungus is excess estrogen unchecked by progesterone. Excess estrogen increases the amount of glucose in the vaginal mucus, which feeds the fungus and allows it to flourish, so yeast infections become more common as we age and start to have anovulatory cycles (Hamad, Abu-Elteen, and Ghaleb 2004; Tarry et al. 2005). This condition can be verified by a vaginal culture. If candida is present, test estrogen and progesterone levels to determine if estrogen is too high relative to progesterone.

Yellowish skin and whites of the eyes: Also called *jaundice*, this yellowish coloration is caused by a buildup of *bilirubin*, a natural pigment, which the body normally disposes of efficiently. There are several reasons jaundice develops, including an underactive thyroid gland, infection, blockages of the bowel or bile duct, and hepatitis. Test levels of thyroid hormones to determine if hypothyroidism is the root cause of this symptom.

APPENDIX B

Blood Levels of Estrogen and Progesterone from Various Products

Product	Dose	Manufacturer	Cmax	Cavg
Estrogen			(pg/ml)	(pg/ml)
Climara patch	0.1 mg/day (buttock application)*	Berlex	174	106
Vivelle patch	0.1 mg/day (buttock application)	Novartis Pharmaceuticals	145 ± 71	104 ± 52
Esclim patch	0.1 mg/day (buttock application)	Women First HealthCare	124 ± 66	74 ± 43
Estraderm patch	0.1 mg/day (abdominal application)	Novartis Pharmaceuticals	Not available	67
Alora patch	0.1 mg/day (abdominal application)	Watson Pharmaceuticals	144 ± 57	98 ± 38
EstroGel gel	0.75 mg/day	Solvay Pharmaceuticals	46.4	28.3
Estrasorb	8.625 mg/day	Novavax	Not available	70.2
Progesterone			(ng/ml)	(ng/ml)
Prometrium (oral)	300 mg	Solvay Pharmaceuticals	60.6 ± 72.5	Not available
	200 mg		38.1 ± 37.8	Not available
Prochieve vaginal gel	90 mg (8%)	Columbia Laboratories	14.87 ± 6.32	6.98 ± 3.21
	45 mg (4%)		13.15 ± 6.49	6.94 ± 4.24

Data taken from FDA approval documents.

* Buttock application gives 10 to 20 percent higher blood levels of estrogen than abdominal application.

Definitions:

Cmax is the maximum peak concentration of a drug in the body after dosing. It indicates whether the drug is sufficiently absorbed to provide a therapeutic response.

Cavg is the average level of the drug in the body.

pg/ml = picograms per milliliter

ng/ml = nanograms per milliliter

Resources

GENERAL INFORMATION AND DOCTOR REFERRALS

The following Web Site has links to referral networks for doctors who are familiar with bioidentical hormones. It also provides current, informative data on a variety of hormonal issues, as well as updates to the information contained in *The Perimenopause & Menopause Workbook*: www.HormoneResource.com

DIRECT-TO-CONSUMER LAB SERVICES

These companies let you order your own blood and urine tests without a doctor. We haven't evaluated these companies, so we can't attest to the quality of their products. It's also important to understand that you should always work with a doctor to correctly interpret your lab results. Some of the companies listed below have doctors on staff who are available to consult with you on your results.

Direct Laboratory Services
P.O. Box 601
Mandeville, LA 70470-0601
800-908-0000
www.directlabs.com

HealthCheckUSA
8700 Crownhill Rd., Suite 110
San Antonio, TX 78209
800-929-2044
www.healthcheckusa.com

Health-Tests Direct
1835 Newport Blvd., Suite D-258
Costa Mesa, CA 92627
800-456-4647
www.health-tests-direct.com

IODINE TESTING

FFP Laboratories
500 South Allen Rd., Suite 1
Flat Rock, NC 28731
877-999-5556

Recommended Reading

Barnes, B. O., and L. Galton. 1976. *Hypothyroidism: The Unsuspected Illness.* New York: Harper & Row.

Brownstein, D. 2002. *Overcoming Thyroid Disorders.* West Bloomfield, MI: Medical Alternatives Press.

———. 2004. *Iodine: Why You Need It, Why You Can't Live Without It.* West Bloomfield, MI: Medical Alternatives Press.

Colborn, T., D. Dumanoski, and J. P. Myers. 1997. *Our Stolen Future.* New York: Plume Books.

Durrant-Peatfield, B. 2002. *The Great Thyroid Scandal and How to Survive It.* London: Barons Down Publishing.

Gillson, G., and T. Marsden. 2003. *You've Hit Menopause: Now What? Three Simple Steps to Restoring Hormone Balance.* Calgary, Alberta: Blitzprint.

Honeyman-Lowe, G., and J. Lowe. 2003. *Your Guide to Metabolic Health.* Boulder, CO: McDowell Health-Science Books.

Jefferies, W. M. 1996. *Safe Uses of Cortisol.* Springfield, IL: Charles C. Thomas.

Lee, J. R., and V. Hopkins. 1996. *What Your Doctor May Not Tell You About Menopause.* New York: Warner Books.

Sapolsky, R. 2004. *Why Zebras Don't Get Ulcers.* New York: Henry Holt.

Schwarzbein, D., and N. Deville. 1999. *The Schwarzbein Principle.* Deerfield Beach, FL: Health Communications.

Sheehy, G. 1992. *The Silent Passage: Menopause.* New York: Random House.

Shippen, E., and W. Fryer. 1998. *The Testosterone Syndrome: The Critical Factor for Energy, Health, and Sexuality; Reversing the Male Menopause.* New York: M. Evans and Company.

Somers, S. 2004. *The Sexy Years.* New York: Crown Publishing Group.

Talbot, S. 2002. *The Cortisol Connection: Why Stress Makes You Fat and Ruins Your Health—And What You Can Do About It.* Alameda, CA: Hunter House Publishers.

Vliet, E. L. 1995. *Screaming to Be Heard: Hormone Connections Women Suspect and Doctors Still Ignore.* New York: M. Evans and Company.

Wilson, J. L. 2001. *Adrenal Fatigue: The 21st Century Stress Syndrome.* Petaluma, CA: Smart Publications.

References

Abdel Khalek, K., M. el Kholy, M. Rafik, M. Fathalla, and E. Heikal. 1991. Effect of triiodothyronine on cyclic AMP and pulmonary function tests in bronchial asthma. *Journal of Asthma* 28(6):425-31.

Abitbol, J., P. Abitbol, and B. Abitbol. 1999. Sex hormones and the female voice. *Journal of Voice* 13(3):424-46.

Abraham, G. E., J. D. Flechas, and J. C. Hakala. 2002a. Effect of daily ingestion of a tablet containing 5 mg iodine and 7.5 mg iodide as the potassium salt, for a period of 3 months, on the results of thyroid function tests and thyroid volume by ultrasonometry in ten euthyroid Caucasian women. *Original Internist* 9:6-20.

———. 2002b. Orthoiodosupplementation: Iodine sufficiency of the whole human body. *Original Internist* 9:30-41.

Abrams, F. R. 1995. The Postmenopausal Estrogen/Progestin Interventions Trial. *Journal of the American Medical Association* 274(21):1675.

Adams, M. R., J. R. Kaplan, S. B. Manuck, D. R. Koritnik, J. S. Parks, M. S. Wolfe, and T. B. Clarkson. 1990. Inhibition of coronary artery atherosclerosis by 17-beta estradiol in ovariectomized monkeys: Lack of an effect of added progesterone. *Arteriosclerosis* 10(6):1051-57.

Aldrighi, J. M., I. N. Alecrin, M. A. Caldas, O. C. Gebara, J. A. Ramires, and G. M. Rosano. 2004. Effects of estradiol on myocardial global performance index in hypertensive postmenopausal women. *Gynecological Endocrinology* 19(5):282-92.

Aloia, J. F., D. M. McGowan, A. N. Vaswani, P. Ross, and S. H. Cohn. 1991. Relationship of menopause to skeletal and muscle mass. *American Journal of Clinical Nutrition* 53:1378-83.

American Association of Clinical Endocrinologists. 2003. Over thirteen million Americans with thyroid disease remain undiagnosed. Press release, January.

American College of Obstetricians and Gynecologists. 2005. No scientific evidence supporting effectiveness or safety of compounded bioidentical hormone therapy. Press release, October 31. Available at www.acog.org/from_home/newsrel.cfm.

American Family Physician. 2000. Uterine fibroid embolization: A new way to treat fibroids. *American Family Physician* 61(12):3611.

Andrew, R., D. I. Phillips, and B. R. Walker. 1998. Obesity and gender influence cortisol secretion and metabolism in man. *Journal of Clinical Endocrinology and Metabolism* 83(5):1806-9.

Ansquer, Y., A. Legrand, A. F. Bringuier, N. Vadrot, B. Lardeux, L. Mandelbrot, and G. Feldmann. 2005. Progesterone induces BRCA1 mRNA decrease, cell cycle alterations and apoptosis in the MCF7 breast cancer cell line. *Anticancer* 25(1A):243-48.

Asthana, S., L. D. Baker, S. Craft, F. Z. Stanczyk, R. C. Veith, M. A. Raskind, and S. R. Plymate. 2001. High-dose estradiol improves cognition for women with AD: Results of a randomized study. *Neurology* 57(4):605-12.

Ballard, V. L., and J. M. Edelberg. 2005. Harnessing hormonal signaling for cardioprotection. *Science of Aging Knowledge Environment* 51:re6.

Barnes, B. O., and L. Galton. 1976. *Hypothyroidism: The Unsuspected Illness.* New York: Harper & Row.

Bixler, E. O., A. N. Vgontzas, H. M. Lin, T. Ten Have, B. E. Leiby, A. Vela-Bueno, and A. Kales. 2000. Association of hypertension and sleep-disordered breathing. *Archives of Internal Medicine* 160(15):2289-95.

Bjorntorp, P., and R. Rosmond. 2000. Obesity and cortisol. *Nutrition* 16(10):924-36.

Boffetta, P., M. Hashibe, C. La Vecchia, W. Zatonski, and J. Rehm. 2006. The burden of cancer attributable to alcohol drinking. *International Journal of Cancer* 119(4):884-87.

Bon, E., Y. Rolland, M. Laroche, A. Cantagrel, and B. Mazieres. 1996. Hypothyroidism on Colchimax revealed by restless legs syndrome. *Revue du Rhumatisme (English ed.)* 63(4):304.

Brabin, L. 2002. Interactions of the female hormonal environment, susceptibility to viral infections, and disease progression. *AIDS Patient Care and STDS* 16(5):211-21.

Brandt, M. L. 2006. Laparoscopic procedure can help to treat infertility. *Stanford Report*, January 18, p. 7.

Bunevicius, R., G. Kazanavicius, R. Zalinkevicius, and A. J. Prange. 1999. Effects of thyroxine as compared with thyroxine plus triiodothyronine in patients with hypothyroidism. *New England Journal of Medicine* 340(6):424-29.

Cakir, M., N. Samanci, N. Balci, and M. K. Balci. 2003. Musculoskeletal manifestations in patients with thyroid disease. *Clinical Endocrinology (Oxford)* 59(2):162-67.

Cali, R. W. 1972. Management of the climacteric and postmenopausal woman. *Medical Clinics of North America* 56(3):789-800.

Carani, C., A. M. Isidori, A. Granata, E. Carosa, M. Maggi, A. Lenzi, and E. A. Jannini. 2005. Multicenter study on the prevalence of sexual symptoms in male hypo- and hyperthyroid patients. *Journal of Clinical Endocrinology and Metabolism* 90(12):6472-79.

Cardozo, L., G. Bachmann, D. McClish, D. Fonda, and L. Birgerson. 1998. Meta-analysis of estrogen therapy in the management of urogenital atrophy in postmenopausal women: Second report of the Hormones and Urogenital Therapy Committee. *Obstetrics and Gynecology* 92(4 Pt 2):722-27.

Carlsten, H. 2005. Immune responses and bone loss: The estrogen connection. *Immunological Reviews* 208:194-206.

Charkoudian, N. 2003. Skin blood flow in adult human thermoregulation: How it works, when it does not, and why. *Mayo Clinic Proceedings* 78(5):603-12.

Chen, A., and D. Huminer. 1991. The role of estrogen receptors in the development of gallstones and gallbladder cancer. *Medical Hypotheses* 36(3):259-60.

Chen, B., D. Zhang, and J. W. Pollard. 2003. Progesterone regulation of the mammalian ortholog of methylcitrate dehydratase (immune response gene 1) in the uterine epithelium during implantation through the protein kinase C pathway. *Molecular Endocrinology* 17(11):2340-54.

Colditz, G. A., B. A. Rosner, and F. E. Speizer. 1996. Risk factors for breast cancer according to family history of breast cancer: For the Nurses' Health Study Research Group. *Journal of the National Cancer Institute* 88(14):1003-4.

Cowan, L. D., L. Gordis, J. A. Tomascia, and G. S. Jones. 1981. Breast cancer incidence in women with a history of progesterone deficiency. *American Journal of Epidemiology* 114:209-217.

Cutolo, M., and A. T. Masi. 2005. Circadian rhythms and arthritis. *Rheumatic Diseases Clinics of North America* 31(1):115-29, ix-x.

Deen, K. I., S. L. Seneviratne, and H. J. de Silva. 1999. Anorectal physiology and transit in patients with disorders of thyroid metabolism. *Journal of Gastroenterology and Hepatology* 14(4):384-87.

Di Giorgio, A., M. Hudson, W. Jerjes, and A. J. Cleare. 2005. 24-hour pituitary and adrenal hormone profiles in chronic fatigue syndrome. *Psychosomatic Medicine* 67:433-40.

Duntas, L. H. 2002. Thyroid disease and lipids. *Thyroid* 12(4):287-93.

Durrant-Peatfield, B. 2002. *The Great Thyroid Scandal and How to Survive It*. London: Barons Down Publishing.

Elliott, B. 2000. Diagnosing and treating hypothyroidism. *Nurse Practitioner Forum* 25(3):92-94, 99-105.

Eriksson, M., N. Egberg, S. Wamala, K. Orth-Gomer, M. A. Mittleman, and K. Schenk-Gustafsson. 1999. Relationship between plasma fibrinogen and coronary heart disease in women. *Arteriosclerosis, Thrombosis, and Vascular Biology* 19(1):67-72.

Eskin, B., and L. Dumas. 1995. *Midlife Can Wait: How to Stay Young and Healthy After 35*. New York: Ballantine Books.

Everhart, J. E., M. Khare, M. Hill, and K. R. Maurer. 1999. Prevalence and ethnic differences in gallbladder disease in the United States. *Gastroenterology* 117(3):632-39.

Fata, J. E., V. Chaudhary, and R. Khokha. 2001. Cellular turnover in the mammary gland is correlated with systemic levels of progesterone and not 17beta-estradiol during the estrous cycle. *Biology of Reproduction* 65(3):680-88.

Fernandez, M., A. Giuliani, S. Pirondi, G. D'Intino, L. Giardinio, L. Aloe, R. Levi-Montalcini, and L. Calza. 2004. Thyroid hormone administration enhances remyelination in chronic demyelinating inflammatory disease. *Proceedings of the National Academy of Sciences of the United States of America* 101(46):16363-68.

Fistarol, S. K. 2002. Skin and hair, marker organs for thyroid diseases. [In German.] *Schweizerische Rundschau für Medizin Praxis* 91(23):1019-28.

Flegal, K. M., M. D. Carroll, C. L. Ogden, and C. L. Johnson. 2002. Prevalence and trends in obesity among US adults, 1999-2000. *Journal of the American Medical Association* 288(14):1723-27.

Fletcher, G. F., G. Balady, S. N. Blair, J. Blumenthal, C. Caspersen, B. Chaitman, S. Epstein, E. S. Sivarajan Froelicher, V. F. Froelicher, I. L. Pina, and M. L. Pollock. 1996. Statement on exercise: Benefits and recommendations for physical activity programs for all Americans. A statement for health professionals by the Committee on Exercise and Cardiac Rehabilitation of the Council on Clinical Cardiology, American Heart Association. *Circulation* 94(4):857-62.

Formby, B., and T. S. Wiley. 1998. Progesterone inhibits growth and induces apoptosis in breast cancer cells: Inverse effects on Bcl-2 and p53. *Annals of Clinical and Laboratory Science* 28(6):360-69.

Furlanetto, T. W., R. B. Nunes, A. M. I. Sopelsa, and R. M. B. Maciel. 2001. Estradiol decreases iodide uptake by rat thyroid follicular FRTL-5 cells. *Brazilian Journal of Medical and Biological Research* 34(2):259-63.

Gapstur, S. M., M. Morrow, and T. A. Sellers. 1999. Hormone replacement therapy and risk of breast cancer with a favorable histology: Results of the Iowa Women's Health Study. *Journal of the American Medical Association* 281(22):2091-97.

Ghent, W. R., B. A. Eskin, D. A. Low, and L. P. Hill. 1993. Iodine replacement in fibrocystic disease of the breast. *Canadian Journal of Surgery* 36(5):405.

Girdler, S. S., C. A. Pedersen, and K. C. Light. 1995. Thyroid axis function during the menstrual cycle in women with premenstrual syndrome. *Psychoneuroendocrinology* 20(4):395-403.

Good, M., M. Day, and J. L. Muir. 1999. Cyclical changes in endogenous levels of oestrogen modulate the induction of LTD and LTP in the hippocampal CA1 region. *European Journal of Neurosciences* 11(12):4476-80.

Gordan, G. S. 1985. Estrogen and bone. Marshall R. Urist's contributions. *Clinical Orthopaedics and Related Research* (200):174-80.

Grady, D., and S. R. Cummings. 2001. Postmenopausal hormone therapy for prevention of fractures: How good is the evidence? *Journal of the American Medical Association* 285(22):2909-10.

Gregoire, A. J., R. Kumar, B. Everitt, A. F. Henderson, and J. W. Studd. 1996. Transdermal oestrogen for treatment of severe postnatal depression. *Lancet* 347(9006):930-33.

Grodstein, F., J. E. Manson, and M. J. Stampfer. 2006. Hormone therapy and coronary heart disease: The role of time since menopause and age at hormone initiation. *Journal of Women's Health* 15(1):35-44.

Gruber, C. J., W. Tschugguel, C. Schneeberger, and J. C. Huber. 2002. Production and actions of estrogens. *New England Journal of Medicine* 346(5):340-52.

Gruber, D. M., M. O. Sator, F. Wieser, C. Worda, and J. C. Huber. 1999. Progesterone and neurology. *Gynecological Endocrinology* 13 (Suppl 4):41-45.

Guszkowska, M. 2004. Effects of exercise on anxiety, depression and mood. [In Polish.] *Psychiatria Polska* 38(4):611-20.

Haggerty, C. L., R. B. Ness, S. Kelsey, and G. W. Waterer. 2003. The impact of estrogen and progesterone on asthma. *Annals of Allergy, Asthma and Immunology* 90(3):284-93.

Hamad, M., K. H. Abu-Elteen, and M. Ghaleb. 2004. Estrogen-dependent induction of persistent vaginal candidosis in naive mice. *Mycoses* 47(7):304-9.

Harrower, H. 1922. *Practical Organotherapy.* Glendale, CA: The Harrower Laboratory.

Hassan, I., K. M. Ismail, and S. O'Brien. 2004. PMS in the perimenopause. *Journal of the British Menopause Society* 10(4):151-56.

Healy, B. 2004. So what to do now ladies? *U.S. News and World Report*, March 15.

Heinrich, A. B., and O. T. Wolf. 2005. Investigating the effects of estradiol or estradiol/progesterone treatment on mood, depressive symptoms, menopausal symptoms and subjective sleep quality in older healthy hysterectomized women: A questionnaire study. *Neuropsychobiology* 52(1):17-23.

Hellermann, J., and G. Kahaly. 1996. Cardiopulmonary involvement in thyroid gland diseases. [In German.] *Pneumologie* 50(5):375-80.

Hertoghe, T. 2006. *The Hormone Handbook.* N.p.: International Medical Books.

Hextall, A., and L. Cardozo. 2001. The role of estrogen supplementation in lower urinary tract dysfunction. *International Urogynecology Journal and Pelvic Floor Dysfunction* 12(4):258-61.

Hickey, M., J. Higham, and I. S. Fraser. 2000. Progestogens versus oestrogens and progestogens for irregular uterine bleeding associated with anovulation. *Cochrane Database of Systemic Reviews (Online)* 2:CD001895.

Hollowell, J. G., N. W. Staehling, W. H. Hannon, D. W. Flanders, E. W. Gunter, G. F. Maberly, L. E. Braverman, S. Pino, D. T. Miller, P. L. Garbe, D. M. DeLozier, and R. J. Jackson. 1998. Iodine nutrition in the United States. Trends and public health implications: Iodine excretion data from National Health and Nutrition Examination Surveys I and III (1971-1974 and 1988-1994). *Journal of Clinical Endocrinology and Metabolism* 83(10):3401-8.

Honeyman-Lowe, G., and J. C. Lowe. 2003. *Your Guide to Metabolic Health.* Boulder, CO: McDowell Health-Science Books.

Hornstein, O. P. 1984. The thyroid gland, the parathyroid gland and the skin. [In German.] *Zeitschrift für Hautkrankheiten* 59(17):1125-26, 1129-32, 1137-43.

Hueston, W. J. 2001. Treatment of hypothyroidism. *American Family Physician* 64(10):1717-24.

Irvine, G. A., M. B. Campbell-Brown, M. A. Lumsden, A. Heikkila, J. J. Walker, and I. T. Cameron. 1998. Randomised comparative trial of the levonorgestrel intrauterine system and norethisterone for treatment of idiopathic menorrhagia. *British Journal of Obstetrics and Gynaecology* 105(6):592-98.

Jabbour, S. A. 2003. Cutaneous manifestations of endocrine disorders: A guide for dermatologists. *American Journal of Clinical Dermatology* 4(5):315-31.

Jasienska, G., A. Ziomkiewicz, P. T. Ellison, S. F. Lipson, and I. Thrune. 2004. Large breasts and narrow waists indicate high reproductive potential in women. *Proceedings. Biological Sciences / The Royal Society* 271(1545):1213-17.

Jefferies, W. M. 1994. Mild adrenocortical deficiency, chronic allergies, autoimmune disorders and the chronic fatigue syndrome: A continuation of the cortisone story. *Medical Hypotheses* 42(3):183-89.

———. 1996. *Safe Uses of Cortisol.* Springfield, IL: Charles C. Thomas.

Jensen, A. A., E. J. Higginbotham, G. M. Guzinski, I. L. Davis, and N. J. Ellish. 2000. A survey of ocular complaints in postmenopausal women. *Journal of the Association for Academic Minority Physicians* 11(2-3):44-49.

Karni, A., and O. Abramsky. 1999. Association of MS with thyroid disorders. *Neurology* 53(4):883-85.

Koenig, H. L., W. H. Gong, and P. Pelissier. 2000. Role of progesterone in peripheral nerve repair. *Reviews of Reproduction* 5(3):189-99.

Kovacs, E. J. 2005. Aging, traumatic injury, and estrogen treatment. *Experimental Gerontology* 40(7):549-55.

Krystal, A. D. 2004. Depression and insomnia in women. *Clinical Cornerstone* 6 (Suppl 1B):S19-S28.

Kushner, R. F., and V. Shanta Retelny. 2005. Emergence of pica (ingestion of non-food substances) accompanying iron deficiency anemia after gastric bypass surgery. *Obesity Surgery* 15(10):1491-95.

Kyllonen, E. S., H. K. Vaananen, J. H. Vanharanta, and J. E. Heikkinen. 1999. Influence of estrogen-progestin treatment on back pain and disability among slim premenopausal women with low lumbar spine bone mineral density: A 2-year placebo-controlled randomized trial. *Spine* 24(7):704-8.

Lando, J. F., K. E. Heck, and K. M. Brett. 1999. Hormone replacement therapy and breast cancer risk in a nationally representative cohort. *American Journal of Preventive Medicine* 17(3):176-80.

Lang, Y., N. Lang, M. Ben-Ami, and H. Garzozi. 2002. The effects of hormone replacement therapy on the human eye. [In Hebrew.] *Harefuah* 141(3):287-91, 312, 313.

Laroche, C. M., T. Cairns, J. Moxham, and M. Green. 1988. Hypothyroidism presenting with respiratory muscle weakness. *American Review of Respiratory Disease* 138(2):472-74.

Laughlin, G. A., and E. Barret-Connor. 2000. Sexual dimorphism in the influence of advanced aging on adrenal hormone levels: The Rancho Bernardo Study. *Journal of Clinical Endocrinology* 85(10):3561-68.

Leonetti, H. B., S. Longo, and J. N. Anasti. 1999. Transdermal progesterone cream for vasomotor symptoms and postmenopausal bone loss. *Obstetrics and Gynecology* 94:225-28.

Leslie, K. S., and N. J. Levell. 2004. Thyroid feeding: A forgotten treatment for psoriasis. *Clinical and Experimental Dermatology* 29(5):567-68.

Lessey, B. A. 2003. Two pathways of progesterone action in the human endometrium: Implications for implantation and contraception. *Steroids* 68(10-13):809-15.

Levine, H., and N. Watson. 2000. Comparison of the pharmacokinetics of Crinone 8% administered vaginally versus Prometrium administered orally in postmenopausal women. *Fertility and Sterility* 73(3):516-21.

Lobo, R. A. 1990. Cardiovascular implications of estrogen replacement therapy. *Obstetrics and Gynecology* 75(Suppl 4):18S-25S.

Lopez-Marcos, J. F., S. Garcia-Valle, and A. A. Garcia-Iglesias. 2005. Periodontal aspects in menopausal women undergoing hormone replacement therapy. *Medicina oral, patología oral y cirugía bucal* 10(2):132-41.

Lowe, J. C. 2000. *The Metabolic Treatment of Fibromyalgia*. Boulder, CO: McDowell Publishing Company.

Manson, J. E., F. B. Hu, J. W. Rich-Edwards, G. A. Colditz, M. J. Stampfer, W. C. Willett, F. E. Speizer, and C. H. Hennekens. 1999. A prospective study of walking as compared with vigorous exercise in the prevention of coronary heart disease in women. *New England Journal of Medicine* 341(9):650-58.

Marieb, E. N. 2001. *Human Anatomy and Physiology.* San Francisco: Benjamin Cummings.

Marks, M. B. 1977. Recognizing the allergic person. *American Family Physician* 16(1):72-79.

Martinez, F. J., M. Bermudez-Gomez, and B. R. Celli. 1989. Hypothyroidism: A reversible cause of diaphragmatic dysfunction. *Chest* 96(5):1059-63.

Martinez, L., J. A. Castilla, T. Gil, J. Molina, J. L. Alarcon, C. Marcos, and A. Herruzo. 1995. Thyroid hormones in fibrocystic breast disease. *European Journal of Endocrinology* 132(6):673-76.

MedicineNet. 2006. Definition of standard of care in MedTerms medical dictionary. Accessed May 29, 2006, at www.medterms.com/script/main/art.asp?articlekey=33263.

Miller, J., B. K. S. Chan, and H. D. Nelson. 2002. Postmenopausal estrogen replacement and risk for venous thromboembolism: A systematic review and meta-analysis for the U.S. Preventive Services Task Force. *Annals of Internal Medicine* 136(9):680-90.

Miller, K. K. 1998. Central hypothyroidism due to pituitary/hypothalamic dysfunction. *Massachusetts General Hospital Neuroendocrine Clinical Center Bulletin* 4(3). Accessed June 2, 2006, at http://pituitary.mgh.harvard.edu/NCBV4i3.htm#Hypothyroidism.

Moggs, J. G. 2005. Molecular responses to xenoestrogens: Mechanic insights from toxicogenomics. *Toxicology* 213(3):177-93.

Morrow, L. B. 1977. Hirsutism. *Primary Care* 4(1):127-36.

Nanda, S., N. Gupta, H. C. Mehta, and K. Sangwan. 2003. Effect of oestrogen replacement therapy on serum lipid profile. *Australian and New Zealand Journal of Obstetrics and Gynaecology* 43(3):213-16.

Nash, J. W., C. Morrison, and W. L. Frankel. 2003. The utility of estrogen receptor and progesterone receptor immunohistochemistry in the distinction of metastatic breast carcinoma from other tumors in the liver. *Archives of Pathology and Laboratory Medicine* 127(12):1591-95.

National Uterine Fibroid Foundation. 2004. Statistics. Accessed April 11, 2006, at www.nuff.org/health_statistics.htm.

Nilsson, M., R. Johnsen, W. Ye, K. Hveem, and J. Lagergren. 2003. Obesity and estrogen as risk factors for gastroesophageal reflux symptoms. *Journal of the American Medical Association* 290(1):66-72.

Ozawa, Y. 2005. Edema in endocrine and metabolic diseases. [In Japanese.] *Nippon Rinsho* 63(1):85-90.

Paganini-Hill, A., and V. W. Henderson. 1996. Estrogen replacement therapy and risk of Alzheimer disease. *Archives of Internal Medicine* 156(19):2213-17.

Pazos-Moura, C. C., E. G. Moura, M. M. Breitenbach, and E. Bouskela. 1998. Nailfold capillaroscopy in hypothyroidism and hyperthyroidism: Blood flow velocity during rest and postocclusive reactive hyperemia. *Angiology* 49(6):471-76.

Pearce, E. N. 2004. Hypothyroidism and dyslipidemia: Modern concepts and approaches. *Current Cardiology Reports* 6(6):451-56.

Pelissier, A. 1998. Menopause, hormone replacement treatment (HRT), stomatologic pathologies. [In French.] *Contraception, Fertilité, Sexualité* 26(6):439-43.

Perez-Ruiz, F., M. Calabozo, A. Alonso-Ruiz, A. Herrero, E. Ruiz-Lucea, and I. Otermin. 1995. High prevalence of undetected carpal tunnel syndrome in patients with fibromyalgia syndrome. *Journal of Rheumatology* 22(3):501-4.

Perno, M. 2001. Burning mouth syndrome. *Journal of Dental Hygiene* 75(3):245-55.

Piccirillo, G., F. L. Fimognari, V. Infantino, G. Monteleone, G. B. Fimognari, D. Falletti, and V. Marigliano. 1994. High plasma concentrations of cortisol and thromboxane B2 in patients with depression. *American Journal of Medical Science* 307(3):228-32.

Pino-García, J. M., F. García-Río, J. J. Díez, M. A. Gómez-Mendieta, M. A. Racionero, S. Díaz-Lobato, and J. Villamor. 1998. Regulation of breathing in hyperthyroidism: Relationship to hormonal and metabolic changes. *European Respiratory Journal* 12(2):400-407.

Polanczyk, M. J., B. D. Carson, S. Subramanian, M. Afentoulis, A. A. Vandenbark, S. F. Ziegler, and H. Offner. 2004. Cutting edge: Estrogen drives expansion of the CD4+CD25+ regulatory T cell compartment. *Journal of Immunology* 173(4):2227-30.

Prior, J. C. 1990. Progesterone as a bone-trophic hormone. *Endocrine Reviews* 11(2):386-98.

———. 2005. Ovarian aging and the perimenopausal transition: The paradox of endogenous ovarian hyperstimulation. *Endocrine* 26(3):297-300.

Punzi, L., P. Sfriso, M. Pianon, F. Schiavon, R. Ramonda, F. Cozzi, and S. Todesco. 2002. Clinical manifestations and outcome of polyarthralgia associated with chronic lymphocytic thyroiditis. *Seminars in Arthritis and Rheumatism* 32(1):51-55.

Pustorino, S., M. Foti, G. Calipari, E. Pustorino, R. Ferraro, O. Guerrisi, and G. Germanotta. 2004. Thyroid-intestinal motility interactions summary. [In Italian.] *Minerva Gastroenterologica e Dietologica* 50(4):305-15.

Putnam, J. 2000. Major trends in U.S. food supply, 1909-1999. *FoodReview* 23(1):8-15.

Raine-Fenning, N. J., M. P. Brincat, and Y. Muscat-Baron. 2003. Skin aging and menopause: Implications for treatment. *American Journal of Clinical Dermatology* 4(6):371-78.

Recober, A., and L. O. Geweke. 2005. Menstrual migraine. *Current Neurology and Neuroscience Reports* 5(2):93-98.

Regier, D. A., W. E. Narrow, D. S. Rae, R. W. Manderscheid, B. Z. Locke, and F. K. Goodwin. 1993. The de facto U.S. mental and addictive disorders service system: Epidemiologic catchment area prospective 1-year prevalence rates of disorders and services. *Archives of General Psychiatry* 50(2):85-94.

Reid, J. R., and S. F. Wheeler. 2005. Hyperthyroidism: Diagnosis and treatment. *American Family Physician* 72(4):623-30.

Reiss, M. 1998. Dysphagia as a symptom of myxedema. [In German.] *Schweizerische Rundschau für Medizin Praxis* 87(18):627-29.

Richardson, R. G. 1973. *The Menopause: A Neglected Crisis.* Queenborough, UK: Abbott Laboratories.

Rosano, G. M., F. Leonardo, C. Dicandia, I. Sheiban, P. Pagnotta, C. Pappone, and S. L. Chierchia. 2000. Acute electrophysiologic effect of estradiol 17beta in menopausal women. *American Journal of Cardiology* 86(12):1385-87, A5-6.

Rosano, G. M., C. M. Webb, S. Chierchia, G. L. Morgani, M. Gabraele, P. M. Sarrel, D. de Ziegler, and P. Collins. 2000. Natural progesterone, but not medroxyprogesterone acetate, enhances the beneficial effect of estrogen on exercise-induced myocardial ischemia in postmenopausal women. *Journal of the American College of Cardiology* 36(7):2154-59.

Rybaczyk, L. A., M. J. Bashaw, D. R. Pathak, S. M. Moody, R. M. Gilders, and D. L. Holzschu. 2005. An overlooked connection: Serotonergic mediation of estrogen-related physiology and pathology. *BMC Women's Health* 5:12.

Rylance, P. B., M. Brincat, K. Lafferty, J. C. De Trafford, S. Brincat, V. Parsons, and J. W. Studd. 1985. Natural progesterone and antihypertensive action. *British Medical Journal (Clinical Research Ed.)* 290(6461):13-14.

Sandyk, R. 1996. Estrogen's impact on cognitive functions in multiple sclerosis. *International Journal of Neuroscience* 86(1-2):23-31.

Sano, M. 2000. Understanding the role of estrogen on cognition and dementia. *Journal of Neural Transmission. Supplementum* 59:223-29.

Sarrel, P. M. 2000. Effects of hormone replacement therapy on sexual psychophysiology and behavior in postmenopause. *Journal of Women's Health and Gender-Based Medicine* 9 (Suppl 1):S25-S32.

Schairer, C., J. Lubin, R. Troisi, S. Sturgeon, L. Brinton, and R. Hoover. 2000. Menopausal estrogen and estrogen-progestin replacement therapy and breast cancer risk. *Journal of the American Medical Association* 283(4):485-91.

Schenker, M., R. Kraftsik, L. Glauser, T. Kintzer, J. Bogousslavsky, and I. Barakat-Walter. 2003. Thyroid hormone reduces the loss of axotomized sensory neurons in dorsal root ganglia after sciatic nerve transaction in adult rat. *Experimental Neurology* 184(1):225-36.

Schlienger, J. L. 1985. Restless leg syndrome due to moderate hypothyroidism. [In French.] *Presse Médicale* 14(14):791.

Schmidt, I. U., G. K. Wakley, and R. T. Turner. 2000. Effects of estrogen and progesterone on tibia histomorphometry in growing rats. *Calcified Tissue International* 67(1):47-52.

Schmidt, P. J., G. N. Grover, P. P. Roy-Byrne, and D. R. Rubinow. 1993. Thyroid function in women with premenstrual syndrome. *Journal of Clinical Endocrinology and Metabolism* 76(3):671-74.

ScienceDaily. 1997. Hyperactivity linked to thyroid hormones. *ScienceDaily*, posted March 12, 1997.

Sheehy, G. 1992. *The Silent Passage: Menopause.* New York: Random House.

Shepherd, J. E. 2001. Effects of estrogen on cognition, mood, and degenerative brain diseases. *Journal of the American Pharmaceutical Association* 41(2):221-28.

Sherwin, B. B. 1985. Changes in sexual behavior as a function of plasma sex steroid levels in post-menopausal women. *Maturitas* 7(3):225-33.

———. 1994. Sex hormones and psychological functioning in postmenopausal women. *Experimental Gerontology* 29(3-4):423-30.

———. 1996. Hormones, mood, and cognitive functioning in postmenopausal women. *Obstetrics and Gynecology* 87 (Suppl 2):20S-26S.

———. 1999a. Can estrogen keep you smart? Evidence from clinical studies. *Journal of Psychiatry and Neuroscience* 24(4):315-21.

———. 1999b. Progestogens used in menopause: Side effects, mood and quality of life. *Journal of Reproductive Medicine* 44 (Suppl 2):227-32.

———. 2003. Estrogen and cognitive functioning in women. *Endocrine Reviews* 24(2):133-51.

Sherwin, B. B., and M. M. Gelfand. 1984. Effects of parenteral administration of estrogen and androgen on plasma hormone levels and hot flushes in the surgical menopause. *American Journal of Obstetrics and Gynecology* 148(5):552-57.

Shifren, J. L., G. D. Braunstein, J. A. Simon, P. R. Casson, J. E. Buster, G. P. Redmond, R. E. Burki, E. S. Ginsburg, R. C. Rosen, S. R. Leiblum, K. E. Caramelli, and N. A. Mazer. 2000. Transdermal testosterone treatment in women with impaired sexual function after oophorectomy. *New England Journal of Medicine* 343(10):682-88.

Siddle, N., P. Sarrel, and M. Whitehead. 1987. The effect of hysterectomy on the age at ovarian failure: Identification of a subgroup of women with premature loss of ovarian function and literature review. *Fertility and Sterility* 47(1):94-100.

Silberstein, S. D. 1992a. Advances in the understanding of the pathophysiology of headache. *Neurology* 42(3 Suppl 2):6-10.

———. 1992b. The role of sex hormones in headache. *Neurology* 42(3 Suppl 2):37-42.

Sinaki, M. 1989. Exercise and osteoporosis. *Archives of Physical Medicine and Rehabilitation* 70(3):220-29.

Singletary, B. K., D. H. Van Thiel, and P. K. Eagon. 1986. Estrogen and progesterone receptors in human gallbladder. *Hepatology* 6(4):574-78.

Sitruk-Ware, R. 2000. Progestins and cardiovascular risk markers. *Steroids* 65(10-11):651-58.

Smith, J. W., A. T. Evans, B. Costall, and J. W. Smythe. 2002. Thyroid hormones, brain function and cognition: A brief review. *Neuroscience and Biobehavioral Reviews* 26(1):45-60.

Stachenfeld, N. S., and H. S. Taylor. 2004. Effects of estrogen and progesterone administration on extracellular fluid. *Journal of Applied Physiology* 96:1011-18.

Staropoli, C. A., J. A. Flaws, T. L. Bush, and A. W. Moulton. 1998. Predictors of menopausal hot flashes. *Journal of Women's Health* 7(9):1149-55.

Staub, J., B. Althaus, H. Engler, A. Ryff, P. Trabuco, K. Marquardt, D. Burckhardt, J. Girard, and B. D. Weintraub. 1992. Spectrum of subclinical and overt hypothyroidism: Effect on thyrotropin, prolactin, and thyroid reserve, and metabolic impact on peripheral target tissues. *American Journal of Medicine* 92(6):631-42.

Sturdee, D. W. 2004. *The Facts of Hormone Therapy for Menopausal Women.* New York: Parthenon Publishing Group.

Tanabe, F., N. Miyasaka, T. Kubota, and T. Aso. 2004. Estrogen and progesterone improve scopolamine-induced impairment of spatial memory. *Journal of Medical and Dental Sciences* 51(1):89-98.

Tanriverdi, F., L. F. G. Silveira, G. S. MacColl, and P. M. G. Bouloux. 2003. The hypothalamic-pituitary-gonadal axis: Immune function and autoimmunity. *Journal of Endocrinology* 176(3):293-304.

Tarry, W., M. Fisher, S. Shen, and M. Mawhinney. 2005. *Candida albicans*: The estrogen target for vaginal colonization. *Journal of Surgical Research* 129(2):278-82.

Tikkanen, M. J. 1996. The menopause and hormone replacement therapy: Lipids, lipoproteins, coagulation and fibrinolytic factors. *Maturitas* 23(2):209-16.

Ting, A. Y., A. D. Blacklock, and P. G. Smith. 2004. Estrogen regulates vaginal sensory and autonomic nerve density in the rat. *Biological Reproduction* 71(4):1397-1404.

Tjan-Heijnen, V. C., E. J. Harthoorn-Lasthuizen, R. M. Kurstjens, and M. I. Koolen. 1994. A patient with postpartum primary hypothyroidism and acquired von Willebrand's disease. *Netherlands Journal of Medicine* 44(3):91-94.

Trombelli, L., S. Mandrioli, F. Zangari, C. Saletti, and G. Calura. 1992. Oral symptoms in the climacteric: A prevalence study. [In Italian.] *Minerva Stomatologica* 41(11):507-13.

Tulppala, M., U. Bjorses, U. H. Stenman, T. Wahlstrom, and O. Ylikorkala. 1991. Luteal phase defect in habitual abortion: Progesterone in saliva. *Fertility and Sterility* 56(1):41-44.

U.S. Census Bureau, Population Division. 2005. Annual estimates of the population by selected age groups and sex for the United States: April 1, 2000, to July 1, 2004 (NC-EST2004-02). Available at www.census.gov/popest/national/asrh.

Vaillant, L., and A. Callens. 1996. Hormone replacement treatment and skin aging. [In French.] *Therapie* 51(1):67-70.

Vexiau, P., and M. Chivot. 2002. Feminine acne: Dermatologic disease or endocrine disease? *Gynecologic and Obstetric Fertility* 30(1):11-21.

Vliet, E. L. 1995. *Screaming to Be Heard: Hormone Connections Women Suspect and Doctors Still Ignore.* New York: M. Evans and Company.

Vorherr, H. 1986. Fibrocystic breast disease: Pathophysiology, pathomorphology, clinical picture, and management. *American Journal of Obstetrics and Gynecology* 154(1):161-79.

Wang, M., and Z. H. Yang. 2002. Role of thyroid hormone in peripheral nerve regeneration. [In Chinese.] *Zhongguo Xiu Fu Chong Jian Wai Ke Za Zhi* 16(3):168-69.

Westphal, S. A. 1997. Unusual presentations of hypothyroidism. *American Journal of Medical Science* 314(5):333-37.

Wilansky, D. L., and B. Greisman. 1989. Early hypothyroidism in patients with menorrhagia. *American Journal of Obstetrics and Gynecology* 160(3):673-77.

Wilson, R. 1966. *Feminine Forever.* New York: M. Evans and Company.

Wise, P. M., M. J. Smith, D. B. Dubal, M. E. Wilson, S. W. Rau, A. B. Cashion, M. Bottner, and K. L. Rosewell. 2002. Neuroendocrine modulation and repercussions of female reproductive aging. *Recent Progress in Hormone Research* 57:235-56.

Witelson, S. F., I. I. Glezer, and D. L. Kigar. 1995. Women have greater density of neurons in posterior temporal cortex. *Journal of Neuroscience* 15 (5 Pt 1):3418-28.

Young, E. A., A. R. Midgley, N. E. Carlson, and M. B. Brown. 2000. Alteration in the hypothalamic-pituitary-ovarian axis in depressed women. *Archive of General Psychiatry* 57(12):1157-62.

Yu, X., R. V. S. Rajala, J. F. McGinnis, F. Li, R. E. Anderson, X. Yan, S. Li, R. V. Elias, R. R. Knapp, X. Zhou, and W. Cao. 2004. Involvement of insulin/phosphoinositide 3-kinase/Akt signal pathway in 17 beta-estradiol-mediated neuroprotection. *Journal of Biological Chemistry* 279(13):13086-94.

Index

A

abdominal weight gain, 185
absolute risk, 160
accidents, 37
acne, 185
Addison's disease, 124
adrenal extracts, 133
adrenal fatigue, 114, 124-127; causes of, 125-126; explanation of, 124; symptoms of, 126-127; treatments for, 132-134
adrenal function tests, 128-131; blood pressure test, 129; lab tests, 130-131; pupil-contraction test, 128-129; white line test, 129-130
adrenal glands, 13, 112-136; alcoholism and, 41; cortisol and, 116-127, 132-133; evaluating problems with, 66-67; hormone imbalances and, 18-19; importance of, 114-116; lab tests for, 130-131; pain felt at, 208; restoring balance to, 135; self-tests for, 128-130; sex hormones and, 115-116; stories related to, 112-114; stress and, 115; testing functioning of, 128-131; thyroid function and, 110-111, 116, 118; treatments for, 132-134
adrenaline, 19
adrenocorticotropic hormone (ACTH), 130, 131

aerobic exercises, 134
aging, premature, 206
alcohol use: adrenal function and, 41, 135; cravings related to, 185-186; insulin production and, 147; personal history of, 40-41
aldosterone, 54, 130, 131
allergies, 186
Alora patch, 168, 219
Alzheimer's disease, 164
American Association of Clinical Endocrinologists, 102
androgens, 13
antibodies, 93-94
anxiety, 186-187
"apple" body type, 175
Armour Thyroid, 92, 105
assertiveness, 179-180
asthma, 187
attention-deficit/hyperactivity disorder (ADHD), 187

B

back pain, 187-188
Barnes, Broda, 92, 105
basal body temperature: lower than normal, 206; testing, 99-100
baseline testing, 20-22
benefits of HRT, 162-164; quality of life and, 168; self-assessment of, 166-167
bilirubin, 217
bioidentical hormones, 5, 156-157; benefits associated with, 162-164; blood levels by product, 219-220; compounded, 169-170; cortisol, 132-133; delivery methods for, 173; dosing levels for, 170-172; estrogen, 158, 162-164, 168-169; FDA-approved, 168-169, 170; progesterone, 158-159, 161, 169; resources on, 221-222; risks associated with, 161-162. *See also* hormone replacement therapy
bladder function, 75, 188
bloating, 198
blood clots, 162
blood pressure: high, 122, 202; low, 129, 207
blood pressure test, 129
blood tests: for ACTH levels, 131; for cortisol levels, 130; for hormone levels, 83-87
body temperature, 99-100, 204, 206
body type: hormone levels and, 22-26, 27; self-assessment exercise, 24; stories related to, 24-26; test determining, 175
bone growth/loss, 74, 163-164
bone health evaluation, 176
book resources, 223-224
bowel problems, 188
brain fog, 188
brain function. *See* cognitive function

breast cancer: alcohol consumption and, 41; family history of, 43; fibrocystic breast disease and, 96, 197-198; hormone replacement therapy and, 162; progesterone and, 74
breast ptosis, 192
breasts: deflated/sagging, 192; estrogen and, 74; size of, 22, 23, 27; sore/tender, 211-212
breathing difficulty, 189
"broken record" technique, 180
bruising, 194
Buck Institute, 3
bugs, sensation of, 197
burning mouth syndrome, 189

C

caffeine consumption, 135
cancer: breast, 41, 43, 74, 96, 162, 197-198; endometrial, 162
Candida albicans, 217
carbohydrates: cravings for, 54; types of, 146
cardiovascular system: cholesterol and, 175, 195; estrogen and, 75; hormone replacement therapy and, 162; progesterone and, 75; symptoms related to, 31
carpal tunnel syndrome, 189-190
cell growth, 75
central hypothyroidism, 44, 94
cervical dysplasia, 190
checklists: family medical history, 45-46; personal health history, 31-35
chocolate cravings, 54
cholesterol: elevated, 195; HRT and, 201; importance of, 21; measuring levels of, 175
chronic colds/illnesses, 190
chronic infections, 190-191
Climara patch, 168, 219
cognitive function: estrogen and, 74, 78; hormone replacement therapy and, 164; problems with, 188-189; progesterone and, 74
cold hands/feet, 191
cold temperature, intolerance of, 204
colds, chronic, 190
complex carbohydrates, 54
compound drugs, 169-170
compounding pharmacies, 169
comprehensive metabolic profile, 176
constipation, 191
corpus luteum, 14
cortisol, 13, 19, 116-127; adrenal fatigue and, 124-127; daily production of, 119-120; excessive production of, 120-121; interactions with other hormones, 116-118; liver function and, 117; low levels of, 124-127; progesterone and, 79; reducing levels of, 121; replacement therapy for, 132-133; stress response and, 115;symptoms of excess, 123; testing levels of, 85, 130-131; thyroid hormones and, 116, 117, 118; weight gain and, 120, 144
cravings: alcohol, 185-186; food, 54, 198-199; unusual, 191

creams, estrogen, 173
Crinone, 169, 173

D

dark circles under eyes, 191-192
dental problems/procedures, 40, 199-200
depression, 192-193
DEXA scan, 165, 176
diabetes, 120, 122, 144, 175, 193, 204
dietary changes, 135
Direct Laboratory Services, 222
direct-to-consumer lab services, 222
dizziness, 193
doctors: referrals to, 221; working with, 176-177, 180
dosing levels for HRT, 170-172
drug use: personal history of, 40-41. *See also* medications
dry eyes, 193
dry skin, 193-194
dyspnea, 189

E

ear problems, 31, 214
early menopause, 194
eczema, 194-195
emotional disorders, 134, 205
endocrine system, 9
endometrial cancer, 162
endometriosis, 195
environmental factors: progesterone levels and, 79; sensitivity to, 196
Esclim patch, 168, 219
Estrace, 169
Estraderm patch, 168, 219
estradiol, 11, 158, 168
Estrasorb, 169, 219
estriol, 11, 158
EstroGel, 169, 219
estrogen, 11; assessing deficiency of, 76-77; balance of progesterone and, 70-71, 87-88; bioidentical, 158, 162-164, 168-169; biological functions of, 74-75; blood levels by HRT product, 219-220; body type and, 22, 23, 27; cognitive function and, 74, 78; decline in levels of, 72-73, 140-141, 143; dosing levels for, 170-172; evaluating imbalance of, 66; hormone replacement therapy with, 158, 162-164, 168-169; hypothyroidism and, 94; menopausal symptoms and, 140-141; relationship with other hormones, 75; self-assessment exercise, 24; symptoms of deficient, 17, 76-77; testing levels of, 84; weight gain and, 74, 143
estrone, 11, 143, 158
exercise: adrenal fatigue and, 133-134; benefits of, 121-122, 134
exophthalmos, 209
eyebrows, thinning, 214
eyes: dark circles under, 191-192; dryness of, 193; problems with, 31, 215; protruding, 209; sun-sensitive, 196-197; yellowish whites of, 217

F

family medical history, 42-47; importance of, 42-44; medical conditions checklist, 45-46; stories related to, 42-43, 44, 91-92; using information from, 47-48. *See also* personal health history
fatigue, excessive, 196. *See also* adrenal fatigue
fats, importance of, 21
fat-soluble vitamins, 21
FDA-approved drugs, 168-169, 170
feet: swollen, 213; tingling in, 214
Feminine Forever (Wilson), 148
fertility levels, 203
FFP Laboratories, 222
fibrocystic breast disease, 95, 96, 197-198
fibroids, 185, 215
fibromyalgia, 91, 198
fingernail problems, 189
fluid retention, 198, 213
follicle stimulating hormone (FSH), 2, 69, 70; testing levels of, 84-85, 141
follicles, 14
follicular phase, 14
food cravings, 54, 198-199
formication, 7, 197
FSH. *See* follicle stimulating hormone
functional hypothyroidism, 94

G

gallbladder problems, 74, 199
gastrointestinal symptoms, 32
gels, estrogen, 173
genital symptoms, 32
Glucophage, 144
goiter, 214
Graves' disease, 108
gum problems, 199-200
gynecological checkup, 174

H

hair: drying and fading of, 141; excessive growth of, 196; loss of, 200
hands: swollen, 213; tingling in, 214
HDL cholesterol, 175
headaches, 200
health history, 28-48; family, 42-47; importance of, 30; personal, 28-42; stories related to, 28-30, 42-43; summarizing, 36-42; symptoms checklist, 31-35; using information from, 47-48
HealthCheckUSA, 222
Health-Tests Direct, 222
Healy, Bernadine, 161
hearing problems, 31, 214
heart: estrogen and, 75; hormone replacement therapy and, 162, 164; progesterone and, 75; symptoms related to, 31, 200-201
heart disease: cholesterol levels and, 195, 201; hormone replacement therapy and, 162, 164; pre-HRT evaluation for, 174-175
heart palpitations, 200-201
heartburn, 201
heat, intolerance of, 204

hemorrhoids, 191
HERS study, 162
Hertoghe, Jacques, 92
high blood pressure, 122, 202
hope, 179
hormone imbalance, 17-20, 49-68; adrenal glands and, 18-19; early signs of, 52-54; estrogen and, 17, 70-78, 87-88; food cravings and, 54; menopause and, 20; perimenopause and, 26; premenstrual syndrome and, 53; progesterone and, 17-18, 70-71, 78-81, 87-88; questionnaire for evaluating, 55-67; stories related to, 49-52, 69-70; testing options for, 82-87; testosterone and, 81-82; thyroid gland and, 18; weight issues and, 142-147
hormone replacement therapy (HRT), 3, 152-180; age at start of, 161; benefits associated with, 162-164; bioidentical hormones and, 156-157, 168-170; blood levels by product for, 219-220; compounded drugs for, 169-170; controversy surrounding, 159-161; cortisol and, 132-133; delivery methods for, 173; doctors and, 176-177; dosing levels for, 170-172; early history of, 160; estrogen and, 158, 162-164, 168-169; family medical history and, 44; FDA-approved drugs for, 168-169, 170; menopause and, 150; personal assessment for, 165-167; preparatory tests/checkups for, 172, 174-176; progesterone and, 158-159, 161, 169; quality of life and, 168; resources on, 221-222; risks associated with, 160, 161-162; story related to, 152-154; summary points about, 178; WHI study on, 155-156
Hormone Symptom Evaluation, 55-67
HormoneResource.com Web Site, 221
hormones: baseline testing of, 20-22; basic information about, 9-10; bioidentical, 5, 156-157; body type and, 22-26, 27; five critical, 10-14; origins of word, 10; testing levels of, 82-87, 174; timeline of changes in, 16
hot flashes, 163, 202-203
HRT. *See* hormone replacement therapy
human papillomavirus (HPV), 190
hypertension, 122, 202
hyperthyroidism, 93, 108-110; assessing symptoms of, 109; explanation of, 108; treatments for, 110
hypoglycemia, 203
hypothalamus, 93
hypothyroidism, 93-98; assessing symptoms of, 96-98; explanation of, 93-94; iodine deficiency and, 95-96; treatments for, 104-108
hysterectomy, 149
hysteria, 20

I

illnesses: chronic colds and, 190; personal history of, 36-37; related to stress, 197

immune system: hormones and, 75; weakness of, 190
infections: chronic, 190-191; urinary tract, 215
infertility, 203
injections, 173
injuries, 37
insomnia, 203-204
insulin, 146-147
insulin resistance, 120-121, 144, 175, 216
intercourse, painful, 208-209
intrauterine device, 173
iodine deficiency: hypothyroidism and, 95-96; iodine loading test for, 103; lab for testing, 222; self-test for, 99
irregular ovulation, 68, 78
irritability, 205
irritable bowel syndrome, 188

J

jaundice, 217
joint pain, 205-206, 212

K

Kennedy, John F., 124

L

lab services, 222
lab tests: for adrenal function, 130-131; for cortisol levels, 130-131; for hormone levels, 83-87, 174; for thyroid function, 100-103
LDL cholesterol, 175
leg pain, 187-188
libido, 142
lipid profile test, 175
lipophilic hormones, 173
liver function, 117, 206
low blood pressure, 129, 207
low blood sugar, 203
luteal phase, 14-15
luteal phase defect, 79
lymphatic system, 134

M

male hormones, 13
Mead, Margaret, 150
medical history. *See* health history
medications: compounded, 169-170; FDA-approved, 168-169, 170; heightened sensitivity to, 201; personal history of using, 41; thyroid replacement, 106. *See also* drug use; hormone replacement therapy
memory: hormones and, 74; problems with, 188-189
menopause, 137-151; early onset of, 194; estrogen deficiency at, 140-141; evaluating symptoms of, 67; experiences of women at, 139; historical perspective on, 148; hormone imbalance and, 20; insulin production and, 146-147; schools of thought about, 149-150; stories related to, 137-139, 147-148; telltale signs of, 141-142; weight gain at, 142-147

menstrual cycle, 14-16; changes in, 206, 210; heavy bleeding in, 210; premenstrual syndrome and, 53, 209
menstrual history, 38-39
mental health. *See* psychological functioning
metabolic syndrome, 120
metabolism: testing for problems with, 176; thyroid hormone and, 90-91, 108
metabolites, 173
migraines, 200
minerals, 133
mittelschmerz, 208
mood swings, 163, 205
morning sluggishness, 211
mouth, burning, 189
muscle weakness, 207
musculoskeletal symptoms, 33
myxedema, 198, 209

N

nasal problems, 31
National Health and Examination Survey, 95
National Institutes of Health, 148, 154, 155
neck, thickening of, 214
nervous system, 75
neurological symptoms, 33
night sweats, 202-203
Nurses' Health Study, 134

O

oral estrogen, 169, 173
oral progesterone, 169, 173
osteopenia, 207
osteoporosis, 165, 207-208
ovarian cysts, 185
ovary pain, 208
ovulation: irregular, 68, 78; pain during, 208; testing for, 78, 83
ovulation self-test, 83

P

pain and stiffness, 212
pale face/lips, 209
panic attacks, 186-187
patches, estrogen, 168-169, 219
"pear" body type, 175
perimenopause, 26, 53
periodontal disease, 199
periods, changes in, 206
personal health history, 26, 28-42; importance of, 30; story related to, 28-30; summarizing with details, 36-42; symptoms checklist for, 31-35; using information from, 47-48. *See also* family medical history
physicians: referrals to, 221; working with, 176-177, 180
pica, 191
pituitary gland, 93
polycystic ovary syndrome (PCOS), 144
Postmenopausal Estrogen/Progestin Interventions (PEPI) Trial, 201

pregnancy: hormones released during, 8; personal history of, 39-40
Premarin, 155, 156, 178
premature ovarian failure, 194
premenstrual syndrome (PMS), 53, 209
Prempro, 153, 155, 178
primary hypothyroidism, 94
Prochieve, 169, 173, 219
progesterone, 12; assessing deficiency of, 80-81; balance of estrogen and, 70-71, 87-88; bioidentical, 158-159, 161, 169; biological functions of, 74-75; blood levels by HRT product, 219-220; decline in levels of, 78-79; dosing levels for, 170-172; evaluating imbalances of, 66; hormone replacement therapy with, 158-159, 161, 169; relationship with other hormones, 75; symptoms of deficient, 17-18, 80-81; testing levels of, 84; weight gain and, 74, 144
Prometrium, 169, 219
protruding eyes, 209
Provera, 154, 155, 156
psoriasis, 194-195
psychological functioning: estrogen and, 75; exercise and, 134; progesterone and, 75; symptoms related to, 33, 212-213
puberty, 10
PubMed, 3, 154
puffy skin, 209
pulse rate, 216
pupil-contraction test, 128-129

Q

quality of life, 168
questionnaire, hormone symptom evaluation, 55-67

R

reactive hypoglycemia, 204
recommended reading, 223-224
referral networks, 221
refined carbohydrates, 54
relative risk, 160
reproductive organs, 74
resources, 221-222; direct-to-consumer lab services, 222; HormoneResource.com Web Site, 221; iodine testing lab, 222; recommended readings, 223-224
respiratory problems, 34
restless legs syndrome, 209-210
reverse T3 (RT3) test, 103
risks associated with HRT, 161-162; self-assessment for, 166-167; statistics related to, 160-161

S

sagging breasts, 192
saliva tests: for cortisol levels, 131; for hormone levels, 85-86
Sarrel, Philip, 142, 149
scalloped tongue, 210
sciatica, 187
secondary hypothyroidism, 94
self-tests: adrenal function, 128-130; iodine deficiency, 99; ovulation, 83

Sergent, Emile, 129
sex hormones, 9, 115-116
sexual desire, 142, 192
sexual function: estrogen and, 75; painful intercourse and, 208-209; progesterone and, 75
SHBG (sex hormone binding globulin), 145, 185
simple carbohydrates, 54
sinus problems, 31, 211
skin: discoloration of, 212, 217; dry and thin, 193-194; hormone replacement therapy and, 164; problems with, 34, 185, 193-194; puffy, 209; yellowish, 217
skin tags, 120
sleep: estrogen and, 75, 143; problems with, 203-204; progesterone and, 75
sluggishness, morning, 211
snoring, 211
Somers, Suzanne, 156
stiffness, 212
stomach upset, 214
stress, 19, 115
stress hormones, 13
subclinical hyperthyroidism, 110
substance use history, 40-41
sugar cravings, 54
sunlight, sensitivity to, 196-197
suppositories, 173
surgeries: hysterectomy, 149; personal history of, 38
swallow test, 99
swollen hands/feet, 213
symptoms, 181-217; adrenal fatigue, 126-127; estrogen deficiency, 76-77; excess cortisol, 123; health history checklist of, 31-35; hormone imbalance evaluation of, 55-67; hyperthyroidism, 109; hypothyroidism, 96-98; progesterone deficiency, 80-81; summarizing with details, 36-42. *See also specific symptoms*
syndrome X, 120

T

T3 hormone, 93, 101-102; replacement therapy, 106
T4 hormone, 93, 101-102; replacement therapy, 105, 106
tertiary hypothyroidism, 94
testing: baseline, 20-22; cortisol levels, 85; estrogen levels, 84; FSH levels, 84-85; HRT preparatory, 172, 174-176; iodine deficiency, 99, 103, 222; laboratory, 83-87, 100-103, 130-131, 222; ovulation self-test, 83; progesterone levels, 84; testosterone levels, 84; thyroid function, 85, 98-104
testosterone, 13, 81-82; deficiency symptoms, 81; excess symptoms, 82; testing levels of, 84; weight issues and, 145
thick tongue, 210
throat problems, 31
thyroglobulin antibodies (TgAb), 103
thyroid ablation, 110
thyroid gland, 93-94

thyroid hormones, 12, 89-111; adrenal glands and, 110-111, 116, 118; cortisol and, 116, 117, 118; evaluating imbalance of, 66; family history and, 44, 91-92; food cravings and, 54; hyperthyroidism and, 108-110; hypothyroidism and, 93-98, 104-108; imbalances of, 18, 89-111; iodine deficiency and, 95-96, 99, 103; metabolism and, 90-91; prevalence of problems with, 92; problems caused by supplemental, 213; restoring balance to, 110-111; stories related to, 89-90, 103-104, 107-108; testing levels of, 85, 98-104; treating imbalances of, 104-108, 110; weight gain and, 90, 145
thyroid peroxidase antibodies (TPOab), 103
thyroid stimulating hormone (TSH), 85, 93; testing levels of, 101-103
thyrotropin receptor antibodies (TRAb), 103
thyrotropin releasing hormone (TRH), 93
timeline of hormonal changes, 16
tinnitus, 214
tongue abnormalities, 210
tooth problems, 199-200
topical gel/cream, 169
transdermal patches, 173
treatments: adrenal fatigue, 132-134; hyperthyroidism, 110; hypothyroidism, 104-108
TSH. *See* thyroid stimulating hormone
twenty-four-hour urine test, 85, 131

U

upset stomach, 214
urinary function: estrogen and, 75; progesterone and, 75; symptoms related to, 32
urinary tract: changes in, 163; infections of, 215
urine tests, 85, 131
uterine fibroids, 185, 215

V

vaginal changes, 163, 208-209, 215
vaginal gel/cream, 173
vaginal pain/itching, 215
vaginal ring, 173
vertigo, 193
vision problems, 31, 215
vitamins: adrenal fatigue and, 133; fat-soluble, 21
Vivelle patch, 168, 219
Vliet, Elizabeth, 171
voice changes, 216

W

waist-to-hip ratio, 22, 175
walking, benefits of, 134
Web resources, 221

weight issues: abdominal weight gain, 185; cortisol and, 120, 144; estrogen and, 74, 143; menopause and, 141-142; progesterone and, 74, 144; role of hormones in, 142-147; testosterone and, 145; thyroid hormones and, 90, 145; weight gain, 185, 216; weight loss, 217
white line test, 129-130
Wilson, Robert, 148
Women's Health Initiative (WHI), 148, 150, 153, 155-156, 162

XYZ

xenoestrogens, 79
yeast infections, 217
yellowish skin, 217

Kathryn R. Simpson, MS, is the CEO and founder of Cerulean Pharmaceuticals, a biotech company that specializes in research on hormones and their roles in health. She is also research director of the Hormone Resource Center in Santa Barbara, CA. She is personally interested in uncovering new therapies to help women dealing with hormone fluctuations or imbalances. Prior to starting Cerulean, she spent more than twenty years in executive positions in biotech and technology firms. She holds a master of science degree from University of Southern California.

Dale Bredesen, MD, is CEO of the Buck Institute for Age Research, the only institute in the U.S. to focus solely on aging and age-related diseases and conditions. The Institute was recently named one of the top five research facilities in the US by the National Institutes of Health. He also works with his coauthor on research in using bio-identical hormones to treat various conditions, including menopause and autoimmune conditions. Dr. Bredesen regularly gives talks and seminars on various topics related to aging and has published almost 150 articles in scientific journals about his work. He has appeared in major broadcast and print media, and has given hundreds of talks to his colleagues at scientific conferences, research facilities, and universities all over the world.

More titles you might enjoy...

only from new**harbinger**publications

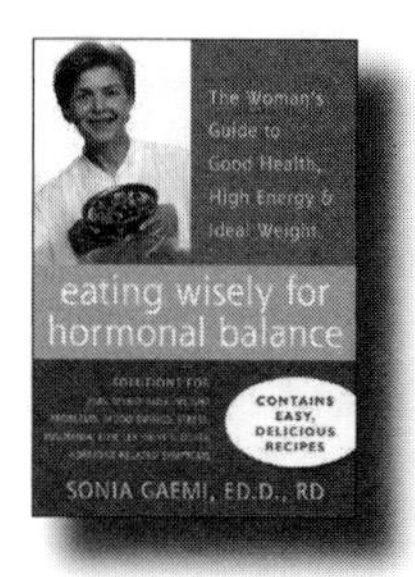

EATING WISELY FOR HORMONAL BALANCE
The Woman's Guide to Good Health, High Energy & Ideal Weight

discover delicious nutritional choices you can make for better health and greater vitality

$16.95 • Item Code: 3732

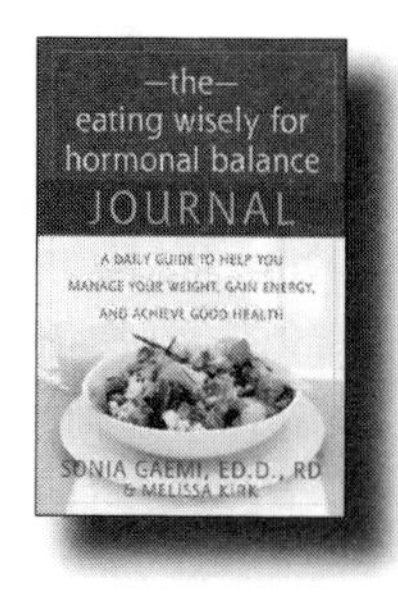

THE EATING WISELY FOR HORMONAL BALANCE JOURNAL
A Daily Guide to Help You Manage Your Weight, Gain Energy & Achieve Good Health

a daily companion and journal to help you make smart and delicious food choices

$15.95 • Item Code: 3945

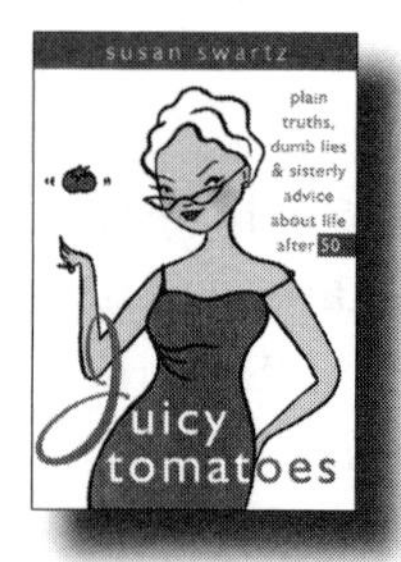

JUICY TOMATOES
Plain Truths, Dumb Lies & Sisterly Advice About Life After 50

women describe the trials and triumphs, in their own words, they experience at age fifty and beyond

$14.95 • Item Code: 2175

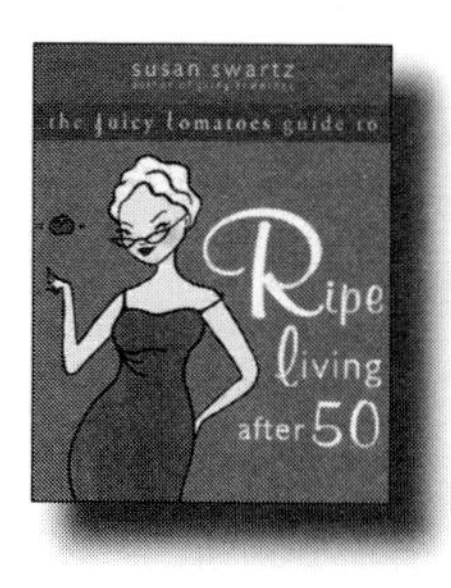

THE JUICY TOMATOES GUIDE TO RIPE LIVING AFTER 50

more first-hand accounts of women's experiences as they wring every drop of juice out of life

$16.95 • Item Code: 4321

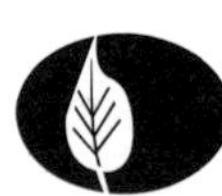

available from new**harbinger**publications
and fine booksellers everywhere

To order, call toll free **1-800-748-6273**
or visit our online bookstore at **www.newharbinger.com**
(V, MC, AMEX • prices subject to change without notice)